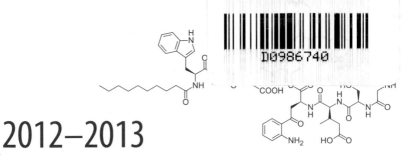

D0986740

2012–2013
Nelson's Pediatric Antimicrobial Therapy

19th Edition

John S. Bradley, MD
Editor in Chief

John D. Nelson, MD
Emeritus

David W. Kimberlin, MD
John A.D. Leake, MD, MPH
Paul E. Palumbo, MD
Pablo J. Sanchez, MD
Jason Sauberan, PharmD
William J. Steinbach, MD
Contributing Editors

American Academy of Pediatrics

DEDICATED TO THE HEALTH OF ALL CHILDREN™

American Academy of Pediatrics Department of Marketing and Publications Staff

Maureen DeRosa, MPA, Director, Department of Marketing and Publications
Mark Grimes, Director, Division of Product Development
Martha Cook, MS, Senior Product Development Editor
Carrie Peters, Editorial Assistant
Sandi King, MS, Director, Division of Publishing and Production Services
Shannan Martin, Print Production Specialist
Linda Diamond, Manager, Art Direction and Production
Kate Larson, Manager, Editorial Services
Kevin Tuley, Director, Division of Marketing and Sales
Linda Smessaert, Manager, Clinical and Professional Publications Marketing

ISSN: 2164-9278 (print)
ISSN: 2164-9286 (electronic)
ISBN: 978-1-58110-654-1
MA0619

The recommendations in this publication do not indicate an exclusive course of treatment or serve as a standard of care. Variations, taking into account individual circumstances, may be appropriate.

Every effort has been made to ensure that the drug selection and dosage set forth in this text are in accordance with the current recommendations and practice at the time of the publication. It is the responsibility of the health care provider to check the package insert of each drug for any change in indications or dosage and for added warnings and precautions.

Brand names are furnished for identifying purposes only. No endorsement of the manufacturers or products listed is implied.

First edition published in 1975.
9-322

1 2 3 4 5 6 7 8 9 10

Editor in Chief

John S. Bradley, MD
Professor of Clinical Pediatrics
Chief, Division of Infectious Diseases, Department of Pediatrics
University of California San Diego, School of Medicine
Director, Division of Infectious Diseases, Rady Children's Hospital San Diego
San Diego, California

Emeritus

John D. Nelson, MD
Professor Emeritus of Pediatrics
The University of Texas
Southwestern Medical Center at Dallas
Southwestern Medical School
Dallas, TX

Contributing Editors

David W. Kimberlin, MD
Professor of Pediatrics
University of Alabama
Birmingham, AL

John A.D. Leake, MD, MPH
Associate Professor of Pediatrics
Rady Children's Hospital
San Diego, CA

Paul E. Palumbo, MD
Director, International Pediatric HIV Program
Dartmouth-Hitchcock Medical Center
Lebanon, NH

Pablo J. Sanchez, MD
Professor of Pediatrics, Division of Neonatal-Perinatal Medicine,
Division of Pediatric Infectious Diseases
University of Texas Southwestern Medical Center
Dallas, TX

Jason Sauberan, PharmD
University of San Diego Skaggs School of Pharmacy
San Diego, CA

William J. Steinbach, MD
Associate Professor of Pediatrics
Assistant Professor of Molecular Genetics and Microbiology
Duke University School of Medicine
Durham, NC

Table of Contents

Introduction

As the diversity and complexity within the field of pediatric infectious diseases increases, it is, of course, impossible for any single person to be proficient in all areas. Previous editions have been supported by contributions from Drs Jason Sauberan in pharmacology, John Leake in tropical medicine, Paul Palumbo in HIV medicine, and Pablo Sanchez in neonatal infectious diseases. We continue this trend in accessing some of the brightest and most practical minds in pediatric infectious diseases in the fields of fungal infections (William Steinbach from Duke University) and viral infections (David Kimberlin from the University of Alabama). While contributions from experts have been made and acknowledged since the first edition of the *Pocket Book of Pediatric Antimicrobial Therapy,* these contributors are now more fully and gratefully recognized as contributing editors. Further, with the success of the digital edition as an "app" for smartphones, and the ability to include references and enhanced commentary on choices of therapeutic agents, the book has evolved from the quick pocket-sized reference to an even quicker, more complete digital reference (although we certainly intend, with American Academy of Pediatrics [AAP], to continue the pocket book format for those, like us, who prefer the feel of a book). To reflect its evolution, we have changed the name of the book to reflect its ongoing metamorphosis as it addresses an important role to provide sound advice in a rapidly changing field: *Nelson's Pediatric Antimicrobial Therapy.* We remain committed to providing practical and evidence-based recommendations to our colleagues who care for children with infectious diseases.

Continuing in this edition, we provide updated assessments regarding the strength of our recommendation and the level of evidence for our treatment recommendations for major infections. In the absence of published high-quality clinical trial data or national guidelines, we use our best judgment from the existing published medical literature, abstract presentations from scientific meetings, consensus statements, and our collective clinical experience. We continue to provide a simplified method to share our evaluations: only 3 categories to rank each recommendation, along with 3 levels of evidence.

Strength of Recommendation	Description
A	Strongly recommended
B	Recommended as a good choice
C	One option for therapy that is adequate, perhaps among many other adequate therapies
Level of Evidence	**Description**
I	Based on well-designed, prospective, randomized, and controlled studies in an appropriate population of children
II	Based on data derived from prospectively collected, small comparative trials, or noncomparative prospective trials, or reasonable retrospective data from clinical trials in children, or data from other populations (eg, adults)
III	Based on case reports, case series, consensus statements, or expert opinion for situations in which sound data do not exist

As has been the case since the first edition, many recommendations in *Nelson's Pediatric Antimicrobial Therapy* fall outside of the US Food and Drug Administration (FDA)-approved indications for children, because many infections are caused by pathogens not evaluated during the initial antimicrobial approval process, many infections occur at tissue sites not originally or subsequently evaluated by the FDA, or drug manufacturers may have decided against applying to the FDA for approval for children for any number of economic or medical reasons. Clearly, the medical literature will often provide us with clinical data, frequently requiring careful interpretation but ultimately providing us with valuable insight. With any drug at any dose, we believe that the potential risks of treatment need to be justified by the potential benefits.

We are particularly indebted to Martha Cook, MS, previously administrative staff manager of the AAP *Red Book* Committee, and currently senior product development editor for the AAP, who has been a remarkable supporter of *Nelson's Pediatric Antimicrobial Therapy* during the past 4 years as we sought to join the AAP family of publications. We thank her for her encouragement, and her discerning insistence that we needed to grade the recommendations and the evidence before we could partner with the AAP! Ms Cook, as well as Jeff Mahony, Mark Grimes, and Maureen DeRosa, continue to be our fully engaged partners at AAP in our shared goal to provide the best care to children.

John S. Bradley, MD, FAAP
John D. Nelson, MD

1. Choosing Among Antibiotics Within a Class: Beta-Lactams, Macrolides, Aminoglycosides, and Fluoroquinolones

New drugs should be compared with others in the same class regarding (1) antimicrobial spectrum; (2) degree of free, nonprotein-bound antibiotic exposure achieved at the site of infection (a function of the in vitro activity for a particular pathogen within the spectrum, the pharmacokinetics at the site of infection, and the pharmacodynamic properties of the drug); (3) demonstrated efficacy in adequate and well-controlled clinical trials; (4) tolerance, toxicity, and side effects; and (5) cost. If there is no substantial benefit in any of those areas, one should opt for using an older, more familiar, and less expensive drug.

Beta-Lactams: Oral Cephalosporins (cephalexin, cefadroxil, cefaclor, cefprozil, cefuroxime, cefixime, cefdinir, cefpodoxime, cefditoren, and ceftibuten). As a class, the oral cephalosporins have the advantages over oral penicillins of somewhat greater safety and greater palatability of the suspension formulations (penicillins have a bitter taste). Cefuroxime and cefpodoxime, which are esters, are the least palatable. The serum half-lives of cefpodoxime, ceftibuten, and cefixime are greater than 2 hours. This pharmacokinetic feature accounts for the fact that they may be given in 1 or 2 doses per day for certain indications, particularly otitis media, where the middle-ear fluid half-life is likely to be much longer than the serum half-life. Cefaclor, cefprozil, cefuroxime, cefdinir, cefixime, cefpodoxime, and ceftibuten have the advantage of adding coverage (to a greater or lesser extent depending on the particular drug) for *Haemophilus influenzae* (including beta-lactamase–producing strains) to the activity of cephalexin; however, ceftibuten and cefixime have the disadvantage of less activity against *Streptococcus pneumoniae* than the others, particularly against the penicillin (beta-lactam) non-susceptible strains. The palatability of generic versions of these products may not have the same pleasant characteristics as the original products.

Parenteral Cephalosporins. First-generation cephalosporins, such as cefazolin, are used mainly for treatment of gram-positive infections (excluding methicillin-resistant *Staphylococcus aureus* [MRSA]) and for surgical prophylaxis; the gram-negative spectrum is limited. Cefazolin is well tolerated on intramuscular or intravenous injection.

A second-generation cephalosporin (cefuroxime) and the cephamycins (cefoxitin and cefotetan) provide increased activity against many gram-negative organisms. Cefoxitin has, in addition, activity against approximately 80% of strains of *Bacteroides fragilis* and can be considered for use in place of metronidazole, clindamycin, and carbapenems when that organism is implicated in non–life-threatening disease. In many countries of the world, cefuroxime has utility as single drug therapy for infants and young children with pneumonia, bone and joint infections, or other conditions in which gram-positive cocci (excluding MRSA) and *Haemophilus* are the usual pathogens. Because of the substantial decrease of *H influenzae* type b (Hib) disease in countries with routine Hib immunization of infants, this advantage in gram-negative spectrum is less important than in the past. However, cefuroxime does retain significant activity against many penicillin non-susceptible strains of pneumococcus.

Third-generation cephalosporins (cefotaxime, ceftriaxone, ceftizoxime, and ceftazidime) all have enhanced potency against many gram-negative bacilli. They are inactive against enterococci and *Listeria* and have variable activity against *Pseudomonas* and *Bacteroides*. Cefotaxime and ceftriaxone have been used successfully to treat meningitis caused by pneumococcus (mostly penicillin-susceptible strains), Hib, meningococcus, and small numbers of infants with *Escherichia coli* meningitis. These drugs have the greatest usefulness for treating gram-negative bacillary infections due to their safety. Because ceftriaxone is excreted to a large extent via the liver, it can be used with little dosage adjustment in patients with renal failure. Ceftazidime has the unique property of activity against *Pseudomonas aeruginosa* that is comparable to that of the aminoglycosides. Ceftriaxone has a serum half-life of 4 to 7 hours and can be given once a day for all infections, including meningitis, caused by susceptible organisms.

Cefepime, a fourth-generation cephalosporin approved for use in children, exhibits the antipseudomonal activity of ceftazidime, the gram-positive activity of second-generation cephalosporins, and better activity against gram-negative enteric bacilli such as *Enterobacter* and *Serratia* than is documented with cefotaxime and ceftriaxone.

Ceftaroline is a fifth-generation cephalosporin, the first of the cephalosporins with activity against MRSA. Ceftaroline was approved by the US Food and Drug Administration (FDA) in December 2010 for adults with complicated skin infections (including MRSA) and community-acquired pneumonia (with insufficient numbers of adult patients with MRSA pneumonia to be able to comment on efficacy). Studies are planned for children.

Penicillinase-Resistant Penicillins (dicloxacillin, nafcillin, and oxacillin). "Penicillinase" refers specifically to the beta-lactamase produced by *S aureus* in this case, and not those produced by gram-negative bacteria. These antibiotics are active against penicillin-resistant *S aureus,* but not against MRSA. Nafcillin differs pharmacologically from the others in being excreted primarily by the liver rather than by the kidneys, which may explain the relative lack of nephrotoxicity compared with methicillin, which is no longer available in the United States. Nafcillin pharmacokinetics are erratic in persons with liver disease. For oral use, dicloxacillin has excellent antistaphylococcal activity in vitro, but is virtually unpalatable.

Antipseudomonal Beta-Lactams (ticarcillin/clavulanate, piperacillin, piperacillin/tazobactam, aztreonam, ceftazidime, cefepime, meropenem, imipenem, and doripenem). Timentin (ticarcillin/clavulanate) and Zosyn (piperacillin/tazobactam) represent combinations of 2 beta-lactam drugs. One beta-lactam drug in the combination, known as a "beta-lactamase inhibitor" (clavulanic acid or tazobactam in these combinations), binds irreversibly to and neutralizes specific beta-lactamase enzymes produced by the organism, allowing the second beta-lactam drug as the active antibiotic (ticarcillin or piperacillin) to bind effectively to the intracellular target site, resulting in death of the organism. Thus the combination only adds to the spectrum of the original antibiotic when the mechanism of resistance is a beta-lactamase enzyme, and only when the beta-lactamase inhibitor is capable of binding to and inhibiting that particular organism's beta-lactamase. Timentin and Zosyn have no significant activity against *Pseudomonas* beyond that of ticarcillin or piperacillin, because their beta-lactamase inhibitors do not effectively inhibit all of the relevant beta-lactamases of *Pseudomonas*. However, the combination does extend the spectrum of activity to include many other beta-lactamase–positive bacteria, including some strains of enteric gram-negative bacilli *(Escherichia coli, Klebsiella,* and *Enterobacter), S aureus* and *B fragilis.*

Pseudomonas has an intrinsic capacity to develop resistance following exposure to any beta-lactam, based on inducible chromosomal beta-lactamases, upregulated efflux pumps, and changes in the cell wall. Because development of resistance is not uncommon during single drug therapy with these agents, an aminoglycoside such as tobramycin is often used in combination. Cefepime, meropenem, and imipenem are relatively stable to the beta-lactamases induced while on therapy and can be used as single agent therapy for most *Pseudomonas* infections, but resistance may still develop to these agents based on other mechanisms of resistance. For *Pseudomonas* infections in compromised hosts or in life-threatening infections, these drugs, too, should be used in combination with an aminoglycoside or a second active agent.

Aminopenicillins (amoxicillin, amoxicillin/clavulanate, ampicillin, and ampicillin/sulbactam). Ampicillin is more likely than the others to cause diarrhea, to disturb colonic flora, and to cause overgrowth of *Candida*. Amoxicillin is very well absorbed, good tasting, and associated with very few side effects. Augmentin is a combination of amoxicillin and clavulanate (see previous text regarding beta-lactam/beta-lactamase inhibitor combinations) that is available in several fixed proportions that permit amoxicillin to remain active against many beta-lactamase–producing bacteria, including *H influenzae* and *S aureus* (but not community-associated MRSA). Amoxicillin/clavulanate has undergone many changes in formulation since its introduction. It is available only in oral form in the United States, but is available for parenteral use in many other countries. The ratio of amoxicillin to clavulanate was originally 4:1, based on susceptibility data of pneumococcus and *Haemophilus* during the 1970s. With the emergence of penicillin-resistant pneumococcus, recommendations for increasing the dosage of amoxicillin, particularly for upper respiratory tract infections, were made. However, if one increases the dosage of clavulanate even slightly, the incidence of diarrhea increases dramatically. If one keeps the dosage of clavulanate constant while increasing the dosage of amoxicillin, one can treat the relatively resistant pneumococci while not increasing the gastrointestinal side effects. Although Augmentin suspensions containing 125-mg and 250-mg amoxicillin/5 mL, and the 125-mg and 250-mg chewable tablets contain the original 4:1 ratio, Augmentin suspensions containing 200-mg and 400-mg amoxicillin/5 mL, and the 200-mg and 400-mg chewable tablets, contain a higher 7:1 ratio. Augmentin ES-600, a suspension formulation of amoxicillin/clavulanate, contains amoxicillin:clavulanate in a ratio of 14:1. This preparation is designed to deliver 90 mg/kg/day of amoxicillin, divided twice daily, for the treatment of ear infections. The high serum and middle ear fluid concentrations achieved with 45 mg/kg/dose, combined with the long middle ear fluid half-life of amoxicillin, allow for a therapeutic antibiotic exposure to pathogens in the middle ear with a twice-daily regimen. However, the prolonged half-life in the middle ear fluid is not necessarily found in other infection sites (eg, skin, lung tissue, joint tissue), for which dosing of amoxicillin and Augmentin should continue to be 3 times daily for most susceptible pathogens.

For older children who can swallow tablets, the amoxicillin:clavulanate ratios are as follows: 500-mg tab (4:1); 875-mg tab (7:1); 1,000-mg tab (16:1).

Sulbactam, another beta-lactamase inhibitor like clavulanate, is combined with ampicillin in the parenteral formulation, Unasyn. The cautions regarding spectrum of activity for Timentin and Zosyn (see Antipseudomonal Beta-Lactams) also apply to Unasyn.

Carbapenems. Meropenem, imipenem, doripenem, and ertapenem are carbapenems with a broader spectrum of activity than any other class of beta-lactam currently available. Meropenem, imipenem, and ertapenem are approved by the FDA for use in children. At present, we recommend them for treatment of infections caused by bacteria resistant to standard therapy, or for mixed infections involving aerobes and anaerobes. While imipenem has the potential for greater central nervous system irritability compared with other carbapenems, leading to an increased risk of seizures in children with meningitis, meropenem was not associated with an increased rate of seizures when compared with cefotaxime in children with meningitis. Both imipenem and meropenem are active against virtually all coliform bacilli, including cefotaxime-resistant (extended spectrum beta-lactamase–producing or ampC-producing) strains, against *P aeruginosa* (including most ceftazidime-resistant strains), and against anaerobes, including *B fragilis*. While ertapenem lacks the excellent activity against *P aeruginosa* of the other carbapenems, it has the advantage of a prolonged serum half-life, which allows for once-daily dosing in adults and children 13 years of age and older and twice-daily dosing in younger children. Newly emergent strains of *Klebsiella pneumoniae* contain *K pneumoniae* carbapenemase enzymes that degrade and inactivate all the carbapenems, reinforcing the need to keep track of your local antibiotic susceptibility patterns. While the current strains are seen predominantly in the Northeast United States, it is not known how quickly or how far these strains will ultimately spread.

Macrolides. Erythromycin is the prototype of macrolide antibiotics. Almost 30 macrolides have been produced, but only 3 are FDA approved for children in the United States: erythromycin, azithromycin (also called an azalide), and clarithromycin, while a fourth, telithromycin (also called a ketolide), is approved for adults. As a class, these drugs achieve greater concentrations in tissues than in serum, particularly with azithromycin and clarithromycin. As a result, measuring serum concentrations is usually not clinically useful. Gastrointestinal intolerance to erythromycin is caused by the breakdown products of the macrolide ring structure. This is much less of a problem with azithromycin and clarithromycin. Azithromycin, clarithromycin, and telithromycin extend the activity of erythromycin to include *Haemophilus;* azithromycin and clarithromycin also have substantial activity against certain mycobacteria.

Aminoglycosides. Although 5 aminoglycoside antibiotics are available in the United States, only 3 are widely used for systemic therapy of aerobic gram-negative infections and for synergy in the treatment of certain gram-positive infections: amikacin, gentamicin, and tobramycin. Streptomycin and kanamycin have more limited utility. Resistance in gram-negative bacilli to aminoglycosides is caused by bacterial enzyme adenylation, acetylation, or phosphorylation. The specific activities of each enzyme in each pathogen are highly variable. As a result, antibiotic susceptibility tests must be done for each aminoglycoside drug separately. There are small differences in comparative toxicities of these aminoglycosides to the kidneys and eighth cranial nerve, although it is uncertain whether these small differences are clinically significant. For all children receiving a full treatment course, it is advisable to monitor peak and trough serum concentrations early in the course of therapy as the degree of drug exposure correlates with toxicity and elevated trough concentrations predict impending drug accumulation. With amikacin, desired peak concentrations are 20 to 35 μg/mL, and trough drug concentrations are less than 10 μg/mL; for gentamicin and tobramycin, depending on the frequency of dosing, peak concentrations should be 5 to 10 μg/mL and trough concentrations less than 2 μg/mL. Children with cystic fibrosis require greater dosages to achieve therapeutic serum concentrations. Inhaled tobramycin has been very successful in children with cystic fibrosis as an adjunctive therapy of gram-negative bacillary infections. The role of inhaled aminoglycosides in other gram-negative pneumonias has not been well studied.

Once-Daily Dosing of Aminoglycosides. Once-daily dosing of 5 to 7.5 mg/kg gentamicin or tobramycin has been used in adults and in some children; peak serum concentrations are greater than those achieved with dosing 3 times daily. Aminoglycosides demonstrate concentration-dependent killing of organisms, suggesting a potential benefit to higher serum concentrations achieved with once-daily dosing. Regimens giving the daily dosage as a single infusion, rather than as traditionally split doses every 8 hours, are safe and effective in adults and may be less toxic. Experience with once-daily dosing in children is still limited, but increasing. In normal children with urinary tract infections, it seems likely that once-daily dosing will become the standard of care; however, for immune-compromised children and for those with other sites of infection, more prospectively collected data are needed before once-daily dosing can be recommended routinely.

Fluoroquinolones (FQs). Based on toxicity to cartilage in weight-bearing joints in juvenile animals investigated more than 30 years ago, pediatric studies were not initially undertaken with ciprofloxacin or other FQs. However, with increasing antibiotic resistance in pediatric pathogens, and an accumulating database in pediatrics suggesting that joint toxicity may be uncommon in humans, the FDA allowed prospective studies to proceed in 1998. As of August 2011, no cases of documented FQ-attributable joint toxicity have occurred in children with FQs that are approved for use in the United States. However, no published data are available from prospective, blinded studies to accurately assess this risk. Unblinded studies with levofloxacin and unpublished randomized studies comparing ciprofloxacin versus other agents for complicated urinary tract infection suggest the possibility of uncommon, reversible, FQ-attributable tendon/joint/muscle inflammation, but these data should be interpreted with caution. The use of FQs in situations of antibiotic resistance where no other agent is available is reasonable, weighing the benefits of treatment against the low risk of toxicity of this class of antibiotics. The use of an oral FQ in situations in which the only alternative is parenteral therapy also represents a reasonable use of this class of antibiotic (American Academy of Pediatrics Committee on Infectious Diseases. The use of systemic fluoroquinolones. *Pediatrics.* 2011;128:e1034–e1045).

Ciprofloxacin usually has very good gram-negative activity (with great regional variation in susceptibility) against enteric bacilli *(E coli, Klebsiella, Enterobacter, Salmonella,* and *Shigella)* and against *P aeruginosa.* However, it lacks substantial gram-positive coverage and should not be used to treat streptococcal, staphylococcal, or pneumococcal infections. Newer-generation FQs are more active against these pathogens; levofloxacin has published, documented efficacy and short-term safety in pediatric clinical trials for respiratory tract infections (acute otitis media and community-acquired pneumonia). No prospective pediatric clinical data exist for moxifloxacin, currently approved for use in adults, although pediatric studies are underway. None of the newer-generation FQs are more active against gram-negative pathogens than ciprofloxacin. Quinolone antibiotics are bitter tasting. Ciprofloxacin and levofloxacin are currently available in a suspension form; ciprofloxacin is FDA approved in pediatrics for complicated urinary tract infections and inhalation anthrax, while levofloxacin is approved for inhalation anthrax only, as the sponsor chose not to apply for approval for respiratory tract infections. For reasons of safety, and to prevent the emergence of widespread resistance, FQs should not be used for primary therapy of pediatric infections, and should be limited to situations in which safe and effective oral therapy with other classes of antibiotics does not exist.

2. Choosing Among Antifungal Agents: Polyenes, Azoles, and Echinocandins

Polyenes. Amphotericin B (AmB) is a polyene antifungal antibiotic that has been available since 1958 for the treatment of invasive fungal infections. Nystatin is another polyene antifungal, but due to systemic toxicity it is only used in topical preparations. AmB remains the most broad-spectrum antifungal available for clinical use. This lipophilic drug binds to ergosterol, the major sterol in the fungal cell membrane, and creates transmembrane pores that compromise the integrity of the cell membrane and create a rapid fungicidal effect through osmotic lysis. Toxicity is likely due to the cross-reactivity with the human cholesterol bi-lipid membrane, which resembles ergosterol. The toxicity of the conventional formulation, AmB deoxycholate (AmB-D), is substantial from the standpoints of both systemic reactions (fever, rigors) and acute and chronic renal toxicity. Premedication with acetaminophen, diphenhydramine, and meperidine is often required to prevent systemic reactions during infusion. Renal dysfunction manifests primarily as decreased glomerular filtration with a rising serum creatinine concentration, but substantial tubular nephropathy is associated with potassium and magnesium wasting, requiring supplemental potassium for virtually all neonates and children, regardless of clinical symptoms associated with infusion. Fluid loading with saline pre- and post-AmB-D infusions seems to mitigate renal toxicity. Three lipid preparations approved in the mid-1990s decrease toxicity with no apparent decrease in clinical efficacy. Decisions on which AmB preparation to use should therefore largely focus on side effects and costs. Two clinically useful lipid formulations exist: one in which ribbon-like lipid complexes of AmB are created (ABLC), Abelcet; and one in which AmB is incorporated into true liposomes (L-AmB), AmBisome. The standard dosage used of these preparations is 5 mg/kg/day, in contrast to the 1 mg/kg/day of AmB-D. In most studies, the side effects of L-AmB were somewhat less than those of ABLC, but both have significantly fewer side effects than AmB-D. The advantage of the lipid preparations is the ability to safely deliver a greater overall dose of the parent AmB drug. The cost of conventional AmB-D is substantially less than either lipid formulation. A colloidal dispersion of AmB in cholesteryl sulfate, Amphotec, is also available, with decreased nephrotoxicity, but infusion-related side effects are closer to AmB-D than to the lipid formulations. The decreased nephrotoxicity of the 3 lipid preparations is thought to be due to the preferential binding of its AmB to high-density lipoproteins, compared to AmB-D binding to low-density lipoproteins-D. Despite in vitro concentration-dependent killing, a clinical trial comparing L-AmB at doses of 3 mg/kg/day versus 10 mg/kg/day found no efficacy benefit for the higher dose and only greater toxicity. Therefore, it is generally not recommended to use any AmB preparations at higher dosages as it will only incur greater toxicity with no real therapeutic advantage. AmB has a long terminal half-life and, coupled with the concentration-dependent killing, the agent is best used as single daily doses. If the overall AmB exposure needs to be decreased due to toxicity, it is best to increase the dosing interval (eg, 3 times weekly) but retain the mg/kg dose for optimal pharmacokinetics. AmB-D has been used for nonsystemic purposes, such as in bladder washes, intraventricular instillation, intrapleural instillation, and other modalities, but there are no firm data supporting those clinical indications, and it is likely that the local toxicities outweigh the theoretical benefits. Due to the lipid chemistry, the L-AmB does not interact well with renal tubules, so there is a theoretical concern with using a lipid formulation, as opposed to AmB-D, when treating isolated urinary fungal disease. There are several pathogens that are either inherently or functionally resistant to AmB, including *Candida lusitaniae, Trichosporon* spp, *Fusarium* spp, and *Pseudallescheria boydii (Scedosporium apiospermum)* or *Scedosporium prolificans*.

Azoles. This class of systemic agents was approved first in 1981 and is divided into imidazoles (ketoconazole), triazoles (fluconazole, itraconazole), and second-generation triazoles (voriconazole, posaconazole) based on the number of nitrogens in the azole ring. All of the azoles work by inhibition of ergosterol synthesis (fungal cytochrome P450 [CYP] sterol 14-demethylation), required for fungal cell membrane integrity. While the polyenes are rapidly fungicidal, the azoles are fungistatic against yeasts and fungicidal against molds. However, it is important to note that ketoconazole and fluconazole have no mold activity. The only systemic imidazole is ketoconazole, which is primarily active against *Candida* spp, and is available in an oral formulation.

Fluconazole is active against a broader range of fungi than ketoconazole, and includes clinically relevant activity against *Cryptococcus, Coccidioides,* and *Histoplasma.* Fluconazole achieves relatively high concentrations in urine and cerebrospinal fluid compared with AmB due to its low lipophilicity, with urinary concentrations often so high that treatment against even "resistant" pathogens isolated in urine is possible. Fluconazole remains one of the most active, and so far the safest, systemic antifungal agent for the treatment of most *Candida* infections. *Candida albicans* remains generally sensitive to fluconazole, although some resistance is present in many non-*albicans Candida* spp as well as in *C albicans* in children repeatedly exposed to fluconazole. *Candida krusei* is considered inherently resistant to fluconazole, and *Candida glabrata* demonstrates dose-dependent resistance to fluconazole. Available in both parenteral and oral (with >90% bioavailability) formulations, clinical data and pharmacokinetics have been generated to include premature neonates. Toxicity is unusual and primarily hepatic.

Itraconazole is active against an even broader range of fungi and, unlike fluconazole, includes molds such as *Aspergillus.* It is available in capsule, solution, and intravenous forms; the solution provides higher, more consistent serum concentrations than capsules and should be used preferentially. Absorption using itraconazole solution is improved on an empty stomach, and monitoring itraconazole serum concentrations is a key principal in management. Itraconazole is indicated in adults for therapy of mild/moderate disease with blastomycosis, histoplasmosis, and others. Although it possesses antifungal activity, itraconazole is not indicated as primary therapy against invasive aspergillosis as voriconazole is now a far better option. Limited pharmacokinetic data are available in children; itraconazole has not been approved by the US Food and Drug Administration (FDA) for pediatric indications. Toxicity in adults is primarily hepatic.

Voriconazole was approved in 2002, but is not yet FDA approved for children younger than 12 years. Voriconazole is a fluconazole derivative, so think of it as having the greater tissue and cerebrospinal fluid penetration of fluconazole, but the added antifungal spectrum to include molds. While the bioavailability of voriconazole in adults is approximately 96%, it is only approximately 50% in children—requiring clinicians to carefully monitor voriconazole trough concentrations, especially in patients taking the oral formulation. Voriconazole serum concentrations are tricky to interpret, confounded by great inter-patient variability, but monitoring concentrations is essential to using this drug and especially important in circumstances of suspected treatment failure or possible toxicity. Most experts suggest voriconazole trough concentrations of 1 to 2 µg/mL or greater. The fundamental voriconazole pharmacokinetics are different in adults versus children; in adults voriconazole is metabolized in a nonlinear fashion, whereas in children the drug is metabolized in a linear fashion. Children require higher dosages of the drug and also have a larger therapeutic window for dosing. Given the poor clinical and microbiological response of *Aspergillus* infections to AmB, voriconazole is now the treatment of choice for invasive aspergillosis and many other mold infections. Importantly, infections with Zygomycetes are resistant to voriconazole. Voriconazole retains activity against most *Candida* spp, including some that are fluconazole resistant, but it is unlikely to replace fluconazole for treatment of fluconazole-susceptible *Candida* infections. However, there are increasing reports of *C glabrata* resistance to voriconazole. Voriconazole produces some unique transient visual field abnormalities in about 10% of adults and children. Hepatotoxicity is uncommon, occurring only in 2% to 5% of patients. Voriconazole is CYP metabolized (CYP2C19), and allelic polymorphisms in the population have shown that some Asian patients can achieve higher toxic serum concentrations than other patients. Voriconazole also interacts with many similarly P450 metabolized drugs to produce some profound changes in serum concentrations of many concurrently administered drugs.

Posaconazole, an itraconazole derivative, was approved in 2006 and is also not currently FDA approved for children younger than 13 years; it is only available in an oral suspension formulation with an intravenous formulation currently in clinical trials. Effective absorption of the currently available oral suspension requires taking the medication with food, ideally a high-fat meal. The pediatric dosing for posaconazole has not been completely determined. The in vitro activity of posaconazole against *Candida* spp is better than that of fluconazole and similar to voriconazole. Overall activity against *Aspergillus* is also equivalent to voriconazole, but notably it is the first triazole with substantial activity against some zygomycetes, including *Rhizopus* sp and *Mucor* sp, as well as activity against *Coccidioides, Histoplasma,* and *Blastomyces* and the pathogens of phaeohyphomycosis. Posaconazole has had some success against invasive aspergillosis, especially in patients with chronic granulomatous disease, where voriconazole does not seem to be as effective as posaconazole for an unknown reason. Posaconazole is eliminated by hepatic glucuronidation but does demonstrate inhibition of the CYP 3A4 enzyme system, leading to many drug interactions with other P450 metabolized drugs. It is currently approved for prophylaxis of *Candida* and *Aspergillus* infections in high-risk adults, and for treatment of *Candida* esophagitis in adults.

Echinocandins. This entirely new class of systemic antifungal agents was first approved in 2001. The echinocandins inhibit cell wall formation (in contrast to acting on the cell membrane by the polyenes and azoles) by non-competitively inhibiting beta-1,3-glucan synthase, an enzyme present in fungi but absent in mammalian cells. These agents are generally very safe as there is no beta-1,3-glucan in humans. The echinocandins are not metabolized through the CYP system, so fewer drug interactions are problematic, compared with the azoles. There is no need to dose-adjust in renal failure, but one needs a lower dosage in the setting of severe hepatic dysfunction. While the 3 clinically available echinocandins each have unique and important dosing and pharmacokinetic parameters, including limited penetration into the cerebrospinal fluid, efficacy is generally equivalent. Opposite the azole class, the echinocandins are fungicidal against yeasts but fungistatic against molds. The fungicidal activity against yeasts has elevated the echinocandins to the preferred therapy against *Candida* in a neutropenic or critically ill patient. Improved efficacy with combination therapy with the echinocandins and other antifungal classes against *Aspergillus* infections is unclear, with disparate results in multiple smaller studies, and a definitive clinical trial is underway.

Caspofungin received FDA approval for children 3 months to 17 years of age in 2008 for empiric therapy of presumed fungal infections in febrile, neutropenic children; treatment of candidemia as well as *Candida* esophagitis, peritonitis, and empyema; and for salvage therapy of invasive aspergillosis. Caspofungin dosing is calculated according to body surface area, with a loading dose on the first day of 70 mg/m^2, followed by daily maintenance dosing of 50 mg/m^2.

Micafungin was approved in adults in 2005 for treatment of candidemia, *Candida* esophagitis and peritonitis, and prophylaxis of *Candida* infections in stem cell transplant recipients. Efficacy studies in pediatric age groups are currently underway, but some pediatric pharmacokinetic data have been published. Micafungin dosing in children is age-dependent, as clearance increases dramatically in the younger age groups (especially neonates), necessitating higher doses for younger children. Doses in children and neonates are generally 2 to 10 mg/kg/day.

Anidulafungin was approved for adults for candidemia and *Candida* esophagitis in 2006. Like the other echinocandins, anidulafungin is not P450 metabolized and has not demonstrated significant drug interactions. Limited clinical efficacy data are available in children; with only some pediatric pharmacokinetic data suggesting weight-based dosing.

3. How Antibiotic Dosages Are Determined Using Susceptibility Data, Pharmacodynamics, and Treatment Outcomes

Factors Involved in Dosing Recommendations. Our view of how to use antimicrobials is continually changing. As the published literature and our experience with each drug increase, our recommendations evolve as we compare the efficacy, safety, and cost of each drug in the context of current and previous data. Every new antibiotic must demonstrate some degree of efficacy and safety before we attempt to treat children. Occasionally, unanticipated toxicities and unanticipated clinical failures modify our initial recommendations.

Important considerations in any new recommendations we make include (1) the susceptibilities of pathogens to antibiotics, which are constantly changing, are different from region to region, and are hospital- and unit-specific; (2) the antibiotic concentrations achieved at the site of infection over a 24-hour dosing interval; (3) the mechanism of how antibiotics kill bacteria; (4) how often the dose we select produces a clinical and microbiological cure; (5) how often we encounter toxicity; and (6) how likely the antibiotic exposure leads to antibiotic resistance in the treated child, and in the population in general.

Susceptibility. Susceptibility data for each bacterial pathogen against a wide range of antibiotics are available from the microbiology laboratory of virtually every hospital. This antibiogram can help guide you in antibiotic selection. Many hospitals can separate the inpatient culture results from outpatient results, and many can give you the data by ward of the hospital (eg, pediatric ward vs neonatal intensive care unit vs adult intensive care unit). Susceptibility data are also available by region and by country. The recommendations made in *Nelson's Pediatric Antimicrobial Therapy* reflect overall susceptibility patterns present in the United States. Wide variations may exist for certain pathogens in different regions of the United States and the world.

Drug Concentrations at the Site of Infection. With every antibiotic, we can measure the concentration of antibiotic present in the serum. We also attempt to directly measure the concentrations in other infected tissues, such as spinal fluid or middle ear fluid. Since free, unbound drug is required to kill pathogens, it is also important to calculate the amount of free drug available at the site of infection. While traditional methods of measuring antibiotics focused on the peak concentrations in serum and how rapidly the drugs were excreted, complex models of drug distribution and elimination now exist, not only for the serum, but for other tissue compartments as well. Antibiotic exposure to pathogens can be described in many ways: (1) the percentage of time in a 24-hour dosing interval that the antibiotic concentrations are above the minimum inhibitory concentration (MIC, the antibiotic concentration required for inhibition of growth of an organism) at the site of infection; (2) the mathematically calculated area below the serum-concentration-versus-time curve (area under the curve, AUC); and (3) the maximal concentration of drug achieved at the tissue site. For each of these 3 values, a ratio of that value to the MIC of the pathogen in question can be calculated and provides more useful information than simply looking at the MIC, as it allows us to compare the exposure of different antibiotics to each pathogen and to compare the activity of the same antibiotic to many different pathogens.

Pharmacodynamics

Pharmacodynamic data provide the clinician with information on how the bacterial pathogens are killed (see suggested reading). Beta-lactam antibiotics tend to eradicate bacteria following prolonged exposure of the antibiotic to the pathogen at the site of infection, usually expressed as the percent of time over a dosing interval that the antibiotic is present at the site of infection in concentrations greater than the MIC. For example, amoxicillin needs to be present at the site of pneumococcal infection at a concentration above the MIC for only 40% of a 24-hour dosing interval. Remarkably, neither higher concentrations of amoxicillin nor a more prolonged exposure will substantially increase the cure rate. On the other hand, gentamicin's activity against *Escherichia coli* is based primarily on the absolute concentration of free antibiotic at the site of infection. The more antibiotic you can deliver to the site of infection, the more rapidly you can sterilize the tissue; we are only limited by the toxicities of gentamicin. For fluoroquinolones like ciprofloxacin, antibiotic exposure is best predicted by the AUC.

Assessment of Clinical and Microbiological Outcomes. In clinical trials of anti-infective agents, most children will hopefully be cured, but a few will fail therapy. For those few, we may note inadequate drug exposure (eg, more rapid drug elimination in a particular child) or infection caused by a pathogen with a particularly high MIC. By calculating the appropriate exposure parameters outlined above, we can often observe a particular value of exposure, above which we observe a very high rate of cure and below which the cure rate drops quickly. Knowing this target value (the exposure breakpoint) allows us to calculate the dosage that will create treatment success in most children. It is this dosage that we subsequently offer to you (if we have it) as one likely to cure your patient.

Suggested Reading

Bradley JS, Garonzik SM, Forrest A, Bhavnani SM, et al. Pharmacokinetics, pharmacodynamics, and Monte Carlo simulation: selecting the best antimicrobial dose to treat an infection. *Pediatr Infect Dis J.* 2010;29(11):1043–1046

4. Community-Associated Methicillin-Resistant *Staphylococcus aureus*

Community-associated methicillin-resistant *Staphylococcus aureus* (CA-MRSA) is a new pathogen in children that first appeared in the United States in the mid-1990s and currently represents 30% to 80% of all community isolates in various regions of the United States (check your hospital microbiology laboratory for your local rate); it is increasingly present in many areas of the world. This new CA-MRSA, like the hospital-associated MRSA that has been prevalent for the past 40 years, is resistant to methicillin and to all other beta-lactam antibiotics, except the newly US Food and Drug Administration (FDA)-approved fifth-generation cephalosporin antibiotic, ceftaroline, for which there are no pediatric data on safety and efficacy (as of August 2011). In contrast to the old strains, CA-MRSA usually does not have multiple antibiotic resistance genes. However, there are an undetermined number of pathogenicity factors that make CA-MRSA more aggressive than its predecessor in the community, methicillin-susceptible *S aureus* (MSSA). Although published descriptions of clinical disease and treatment of the old *S aureus* found in textbooks, the medical literature, and older editions of *Nelson's Pediatric Antimicrobial Therapy* remain accurate for MSSA, CA-MRSA seems to cause greater tissue necrosis, an increased host inflammatory response, an increased rate of complications, and an increased rate of recurrent infections compared with MSSA. Response to therapy with non–beta-lactam antibiotics seems to be delayed, and it is unknown whether the longer courses of alternative agents that seem to be needed for clinical cure are due to a hardier, better-adapted pathogen, or whether alternative agents are not as effective as beta lactam agents against MSSA.

Therapy for CA-MRSA

Vancomycin (intravenous [IV]) has been the mainstay of parenteral therapy of MRSA infections for the past 4 decades and continues to have activity against more than 98% of strains isolated from children. A few cases of intermediate resistance and heteroresistance have been reported, most commonly in adults who are receiving long-term therapy or who have received multiple exposures to vancomycin. Unfortunately, the response to therapy using standard vancomycin dosing of 40 mg/kg/day in the treatment of the new CA-MRSA strains has not been as predictably good as in the past. Increasingly, data in adults suggest that serum trough concentrations of vancomycin in treating serious CA-MRSA infections should be kept in the range of 15 to 20 µg/mL, which frequently causes toxicity in adults. For children, serum trough concentrations of 15 to 20 µg/mL can usually be achieved using the old pediatric "meningitis dosage" of vancomycin of 60 mg/kg/day. Although no prospectively collected data are available, it appears that this dosage in children is reasonably effective and not associated with the degree of nephrotoxicity observed in adults. For vancomycin, the area under the curve/minimum inhibitory concentration (MIC) ratios that best predict a successful outcome are those of about 400 and greater, which is achievable for CA-MRSA strains with in vitro MIC values of 1 or 2 µg/mL. Strains with MIC values of 4 µg/mL or greater should generally be considered resistant to vancomycin. At the higher "meningitis" treatment dosage, one needs to follow renal function for the development of toxicity.

Clindamycin (oral [PO] or IV) is active against approximately 90% of strains, with great geographic variability (again, check with your hospital laboratory). The dosage for moderate to severe infections is 30 to 40 mg/kg/day, in 3 divided doses, using the same mg/kg dose PO or IV. Clindamycin is not as bactericidal as vancomycin, but gets into abscesses better than vancomycin. Some CA-MRSA strains are susceptible to clindamycin on initial testing, but have inducible clindamycin resistance that is usually assessed by the D-test. Within each population of these CA-MRSA organisms, a rare organism will have a mutation that allows for constant (rather than induced) resistance. Although still somewhat controversial for infections that have a relatively low organism load (cellulitis, small abscesses) and are unlikely to contain these mutants, clindamycin should be effective therapy. Infections with a high organism load (empyema) may have a greater risk of failure against strains positive on a D-test (as the likelihood of having a few truly resistant organisms is greater, given the greater numbers of organisms), and clindamycin should not be used as the preferred agent.

Clindamycin is used to treat most CA-MRSA infections that are not life-threatening, and if the child responds, therapy can be switched from IV to PO (although the oral solution is not very well tolerated). *Clostridium difficile* enterocolitis is a concern as a clindamycin-associated complication; however, despite a great increase in the use of clindamycin in children during the past decade, there are no recent published reports on any clinically significant increase in the rate of this complication in children.

Trimethoprim/sulfamethoxazole (PO, IV), Bactrim/Septra, is active against CA-MRSA in vitro and has been used successfully to treat CA-MRSA skin infections by the oral route. There are no prospective comparative data on treatment of skin or skin structure infections, although some retrospective data in children suggest efficacy. Given our lack of information, this antibiotic should not be used to treat more serious infections.

Linezolid, Zyvox (PO, IV), active against virtually 100% of CA-MRSA strains, is another reasonable alternative but is considered bacteriostatic, and has relatively frequent hematologic toxicity (neutropenia, thrombocytopenia) and some infrequent neurologic toxicity (peripheral neuropathy, optic neuritis), particularly when used for courses of 2 weeks or longer (a complete blood cell count should be checked every week or two in children receiving prolonged linezolid therapy).

Daptomycin (IV), FDA approved for adults for skin infections and bacteremia/endocarditis, is a new class of antibiotic, a lipopeptide, and is highly bactericidal against MRSA by causing bacterial cell membrane depolarization. Daptomycin should be considered for treatment in failures with other better studied antibiotics, and may not be effective in the treatment of community-acquired pneumonia due to binding of the drug to surfactant in the lung. Pediatric studies for skin infections are underway.

Tigecycline and fluoroquinolones, both of which may show in vitro activity, are not generally recommended for children if other agents are available and are tolerated, due to potential toxicity issues for children with tetracyclines and fluoroquinolones.

Ceftaroline, a newly FDA-approved cephalosporin antibiotic for adults for skin and skin structure infections (including CA-MRSA) and community-acquired pneumonia, is the first beta-lactam antibiotic to have been chemically modified to be able to bind to the altered protein (PBP2a) that confers resistance to all other beta-lactams. The gram-negative coverage is similar to cefotaxime, with no activity against *Pseudomonas*. As of August 2011, no published data exist for children, except for single-dose pharmacokinetics in 7 adolescents, but a complete evaluation in children is planned. The efficacy and toxicity profile in adults is what one would expect from most cephalosporins.

Combination therapy for serious infections, with vancomycin and rifampin (for deep abscesses), or vancomycin and gentamicin (for bacteremia) is often used, but no data exist on improved efficacy over single antibiotic therapy. Some experts use vancomycin and clindamycin in combination, particularly for children with a toxic-shock clinical presentation (with clindamycin, a ribosomal agent, theoretically decreasing toxin production more quickly than vancomycin), but no data are currently available to compare one antibiotic against another for CA-MRSA, let alone one combination against another.

In Chapter 6, recommendations for treatment of staphylococcal infections are given for 2 situations: standard (eg, MSSA) and CA-MRSA. Cultures should be obtained whenever possible. If cultures demonstrate MSSA, then CA-MRSA antibiotics can be discontinued, continuing with the preferred beta-lactam agents. Rapid tests are becoming available to allow for identification of CA-MRSA within a few hours of obtaining a sample, rather than taking 1 to 3 days for the culture report.

Life-threatening and Serious Infections. If any CA-MRSA is present in your community, empiric therapy for presumed staphylococcal infections that are either life-threatening or infections for which any risk of failure is unacceptable (eg, meningitis) should follow the recommendations for CA-MRSA and include high-dose vancomycin, clindamycin, or linezolid. As beta-lactam antibiotics are considered better antibiotics for MSSA infections, nafcillin or oxacillin should be used in combination with a CA-MRSA–active antibiotic until culture results are available.

Moderate Infections. If you live in a location with greater than 10% methicillin resistance, consider using the CA-MRSA recommendations for hospitalized children with presumed staphylococcal infections of any severity, and start empiric therapy with clindamycin (usually active against >90% of CA-MRSA), vancomycin, or linezolid IV. Standard empiric therapy can still be used for less severe infections in these regions, realizing that a certain low percentage of children who are actually infected by CA-MRSA may fail standard therapy.

In skin and skin structure abscesses, drainage of the abscess seems to be completely curative in some children, and antibiotics may not be necessary following incision and drainage.

Mild Infections. For nonserious, presumed staphylococcal infections in regions with significant CA-MRSA, empiric topical therapy with either mupirocin (Bactroban) or retapamulin (Altabax) ointment, or oral therapy with trimethoprim/sulfamethoxazole or clindamycin are preferred. For older children, doxycycline and minocycline are also options based on limited data in adults. Again, using standard empiric therapy with erythromycins, oral cephalosporins, or amoxicillin/clavulanate may be acceptable in areas with a low prevalence of CA-MRSA and a high likelihood of MSSA as the local staphylococcal pathogen, for which these antimicrobials are usually effective.

Recurrent Infections. For children with problematic, recurrent infections, no well-studied prospectively collected data provide a solution. Bleach baths (one-half cup of bleach in one-quarter filled bathtub) seem to be able to transiently decrease the numbers of colonizing organisms. Bathing with chlorhexidine (Hibiclens, a preoperative antibacterial skin disinfectant) daily or a few times each week should provide topical anti-MRSA activity for several hours following a bath. Nasal mupirocin ointment (Bactroban) designed to eradicate colonization may also be used. All of these measures have advantages and disadvantages and need to be used together with environment measures (eg, washing towels frequently, using hand sanitizers, not sharing items of clothing). Helpful advice can be found on the Centers for Disease Control and Prevention Web site at www.cdc.gov/mrsa/.

The Future. A number of new antibiotics are in clinical trials for adults, including a number of oxazolidinones, glycopeptides, and lipopeptides that have advantages over currently approved drugs in either activity, safety, or dosing regimens. It will be important to see how these drugs perform in adults before recommending them for children. Vaccines against staphylococcal infections have not been successful to date. Immune globulin and antibody products with activity against CA-MRSA are also under investigation.

5. Antimicrobial Therapy for Newborns

NOTES

- Prospectively collected data in newborns are slowly becoming available. In situations of inadequate data, suggested doses are based on efficacy, safety, and pharmacologic data from older children or adults. These may not account for the effect of developmental changes (effect of ontogeny) on drug metabolism that occur during early infancy and among premature and full-term infants. These values may vary widely, particularly for the unstable premature infant. Oral convalescent therapy for neonatal infections has not been well studied, but may be used cautiously in non–life-threatening infections, in adherent families with ready access to medical care.

- The recommended antibiotic dosages and intervals of administration are given in the tables at the end of this chapter.

- **Adverse drug reaction:** Neonates should not receive IV ceftriaxone while receiving IV calcium-containing products including parenteral nutrition by the same or different infusion lines as fatal reactions with ceftriaxone-calcium precipitates in lungs and kidneys in neonates have occurred. There are no data on interactions between IV ceftriaxone and oral calcium-containing products or between intramuscular ceftriaxone and IV or oral calcium-containing products. Current information is available on the FDA Web site. Cefotaxime is preferred over ceftriaxone for neonates with hyperbilirubinemia.

- **Abbreviations:** ABLC, lipid complex amphotericin; AmB, amphotericin B; amox/clav, amoxicillin/clavulanate; AOM, acute otitis media; bid, twice daily; BSA, body surface area; CA, chronologic age; CBC, complete blood cell count; CLD, chronic lung disease; CMV, cytomegalovirus; CNS, central nervous system; CSF, cerebrospinal fluid; div, divided; ESBL, extended spectrum beta-lactamase; FDA, US Food and Drug Administration; GA, gestational age; GBS, group B streptococcus; GI, gastrointestinal; G-CSF, granulocyte colony stimulating factor; HSV, herpes simplex virus; ID, infectious diseases; IM, intramuscular; IV, intravenous; IVIG, intravenous immune globulin; L-AmB, liposomal AmB; MRSA, methicillin-resistant *Staphylococcus aureus;* MSSA, methicillin-susceptible *S aureus;* NEC, necrotizing enterocolitis; NICU, neonatal intensive care unit; NVP, nevirapine; oxacillin/nafcillin, oxacillin or nafcillin; PCR, polymerase chain reaction; pip/tazo, piperacillin/tazobactam; PO, orally; RPR, rapid plasma reagin; RSV, respiratory syncytial virus; ticar/clav, ticarcillin/clavulanate; tid, 3 times daily; TIG, tetanus immune globulin; TMP/SMX, trimethoprim/sulfamethoxazole; UTI, urinary tract infection; VCUG, voiding cystourethrogram; VDRL, Venereal Disease Research Laboratories; ZDV, zidovudine.

A. RECOMMENDED THERAPY FOR SELECTED NEWBORN CONDITIONS

Condition	Therapy (evidence grade) See Table 5B for Neonatal Dosages	Comments
Conjunctivitis		
– Chlamydial	Azithromycin PO for 5 days (AII) or erythromycin ethylsuccinate PO for 10–14 days (AII)	Macrolides PO preferred to prevent development of pneumonia; association of erythromycin and pyloric stenosis in young infants Alternatives: Oral sulfonamides may be used after the immediate neonatal period for infants who do not tolerate erythromycin.
– Gonococcal	Ceftriaxone 25–50 mg/kg (max 125 mg) IV, IM once (AI) (longer treatment may be used for severe cases)	Saline irrigation of eyes Alternative: cefotaxime may be used in infants with hyperbilirubinemia. Evaluate for chlamydial infection. All infants born to mothers with untreated gonococcal infection (regardless of symptoms) require therapy.
– S aureus	Topical therapy sufficient for mild S aureus cases (AII), but oral or IV therapy may be considered for moderate to severe conjunctivitis MSSA: oxacillin/nafcillin IV or cefazolin (for non-CNS infections) IM, IV for 7 days MRSA: vancomycin IV or clindamycin IV, PO	Neomycin or erythromycin (BIII) ophthalmic drops or ointment No prospective data for MRSA conjunctivitis (BIII) Cephalexin PO for mild-moderate disease caused by MSSA Increasing S aureus resistance with ciprofloxacin/ levofloxacin ophthalmic formulations (AII)
– Pseudomonas aeruginosa	Ceftazidime IM, IV AND tobramycin IM, IV for 7–10 days (alternatives: pip/tazo, cefepime, or meropenem) (BIII)	Aminoglycoside or polymyxin B-containing ophthalmic drops or ointment as adjunctive therapy
– Other gram-negative	Aminoglycoside or polymyxin B-containing ophthalmic drops or ointment if mild (AII) Systemic therapy if moderate to severe, or unresponsive to topical therapy (AIII)	Duration of therapy dependent on clinical course and may be as short as 5 days if clinically resolved.

Cytomegalovirus

– Congenital	Ganciclovir 12 mg/kg/day IV d v q12h for 6 wk (AII); or oral valganciclovir to achieve peaks 4–6 µg/mL and troughs of 1 µg/mL (AUC₁₂ of 27 mg·h/L).	Benefit for hearing loss (AII) Treatment recommended only for neonates with CNS involvement. Neutropenia in up to 20%–68% of infants on long-term therapy (responds to G-CSF or discontinuation of therapy) Treatment for congenital CMV should start within the first month of life. CMV-IVIG not recommended
– Acquired	Ganciclovir 12 mg/kg/day IV d v q12h for 14–21 days (AIII)	Only recommended for acute severe disease with pneumonia, hepatitis, encephalitis, or persistent thrombocytopenia. Observe for possible relapse after completion of therapy (AIII).

Fungal infections (see Chapter 8)

– Candidiasis	L-AmB/ABLC (3–5 mg/kg/day) or AmB-D (1 mg/kg/day). If urinary tract involvement is excluded, then can use L-AmB/ABLC due to theoretical concerns. For susceptible strains, fluconazole is usually effective. Load with 25 mg/day, then continue with 12 mg/kg/day (BI). For prophylaxis, fluconazole 3–6 mg/kg/day twice a week in high-risk neonates (birth weight <1,000 g) in centers where incidence of disease is high.	Prompt removal of all catheters essential (AII) Evaluate for other sites: CSF analysis, cardiac echo, abdominal ultrasound to include bladder; retinal eye exam Persistent disease requires evaluation of catheter removal or search for disseminated sites. Antifungal susceptibility is suggested with persistent disease. (Candida krusei inherently resistant to fluconazole. Candida parapsilosis may be less susceptible to echinocandins in candidiasis. Change from amphotericin B or fluconazole to micafungin/caspofungin if cultures persistently positive (BII). Role of flucytosine (5-FC) orally in neonates with Candida meningitis is not well defined and not routinely recommended due to toxicity concerns Length of therapy dependent on disease (BIII), usually 3 wk Limited data exist on echinocandins for meningitis. Higher doses may be needed in the smallest infants. Echinocandins are under investigation, but may not be effective for meningitis or higher doses may be needed. Antifungal bladder washes not indicated.

A. RECOMMENDED THERAPY FOR SELECTED NEWBORN CONDITIONS (cont)

Condition	Therapy (evidence grade) See Table 5B for Neonatal Dosages	Comments
Fungal infections (see Chapter 8) (cont)		
– Aspergillosis (usually cutaneous infection with systemic dissemination)	Voriconazole (18 mg/kg/day divided q12h load, then continue with 16 mg/kg/day. Very important to follow serum concentrations). Duration depends on severity of disease and success of local debridement (BIII).	Aggressive antifungal therapy, early debridement of skin lesions (AIII)
Gastrointestinal infections		
– NEC or peritonitis secondary to bowel rupture	Ampicillin IV AND gentamicin IM, IV for ≥10 days (AII) Alternatives: pip/tazo AND gentamicin (AII); ceftazidime/cefotaxime AND genetamicin ± metroniddazole (BIII); OR meropenem (BI)	Surgical drainage (AII) Definitive antibiotic therapy based on culture results (aerobic, anaerobic, and fungal); meropenem or cefepime if ceftazidime-resistant gram-negative bacilli isolated. Vancomycin rather than ampicillin if MRSA prevalent. *Bacteroides* not common until several weeks of age (AIII). Duration of therapy dependent on clinical response and risk of persisting intra-abdominal abscess (AIII) Probiotics may prevent NEC in infants born <1,500 g but agent, dose, and safety not fully known
– *Salmonella*	Ampicillin IM, IV (if susceptible) OR cefotaxime IM, IV for 7–10 days (AII)	Observe for focal complications (meningitis, arthritis, etc) (AIII)
Herpes simplex infection		
– CNS and disseminated disease	Acyclovir IV for 21 days (AII)	For CNS disease, perform CSF HSV PCR near end of 21 days of therapy and continue acyclovir until PCR negative Foscarnet for acyclovir-resistant disease Acyclovir PO (300 mg/m²/dose tid) suppression for 6 mo recommended following parenteral therapy (AI) Monitor for neutropenia during suppressive therapy.

– Skin, eye, or mouth disease	Acyclovir IV for 14 days (AII) (if eye disease present, ADD topical trifluridine ophthalmic solution OR topical 0.1% iododeoxyuridine) Obtain CSF PCR for HSV to assess for CNS infection.	Acyclovir PO (300 mg/m²/dose tid) suppression for 6 mo recommended following parenteral therapy (AI). Monitor for neutropenia during suppressive therapy. For recurrent cutaneous disease, oral acyclovir until lesions crusted (assuming CNS disease at the time of cutaneous recurrence).
Human immunodeficiency virus infection	Peripartum presumptive therapy and management: ZDV for the first 4–6 wk of age (AI) GA ≥35 wk: ZDV 8 mg/kg/day PO div bid OR 6 mg/kg/day IV div q6h for 6 wk GA <35 wk but >30 wk: ZDV 3 mg/kg/day IV (OR 4 mg/kg/day PO) div q12h. Increase at 2 wk of age to 6 mg/kg/day (4.5 mg/kg/d IV) div q8h. GA <30 wk: ZDV 3 mg/kg/day IV (OR 4 mg/kg/cay PO) div q12h. Increase at 4 wk of age to 6 mg/kg/day PO (OR 4.5 mg/kg/day IV) div q8h. Consider (ir consultation with a pediatric HIV specialist) combination therapies for infants born to mothers who did not receive antepartum therapy or mothers with drug-resistant HIV.	For detailed information: http://aidsinfo.nih.gov/Guidelines Start therapy at 6–8 h of age if possible (AII). Monitor CBC at birth and 4 wk (AII). Some experts consider the use of ZDV in combination with other antiretroviral drugs in certain situations (eg, mothers with minimal intervention before delivery, has high viral load, and with known resistant virus). Since optimal prophylactic regimens have not been formally established, consultation with a pediatric HIV specialist is recommended (BIII). Perform HIV-1 DNA PCR or RNA assays at 14–21 days, 1–2 mo, and 4–6 mo (AI). Initiate prophylaxis for pneumocystis pneumonia at 6 wk of age if HIV infection not yet excluded (AII).
Influenza A and B viruses	Term neonates from birth to 3 mo: treatment: 6 mg/kg/day PO bid for 5 days Prophylaxis is not recommended unless situation judged critical because of limited data on safety/efficacy in this age group.	Current weight-based dosing recommendations are not intended for preterm infants. Preterm infants have more variable, slower clearance of oseltamivir because of immature renal function. Limited data suggest a dose of 2 mg/kg/day PO bid for preterm infants. No duration investigated; follow clinically and by serial respiratory tract PCR test to determine clearing of influenza virus.

A. RECOMMENDED THERAPY FOR SELECTED NEWBORN CONDITIONS (cont)

Condition	Therapy (evidence grade) See Table 5B for Neonatal Dosages	Comments
Omphalitis and funisitis		
– Empiric therapy for omphalitis and necrotizing funisitis direct therapy against coliform bacilli, *S aureus* (consider MRSA), and anaerobes	Cefotaxime OR gentamicin, AND clindamycin for ≥10 days (AII)	Need to culture to direct therapy Alternatives for coliform coverage if resistance likely: cefepime, meropenem For suspect MRSA: add vancomycin Alternatives for combined MSSA and anaerobic coverage: pip/tazo, or ticar/clav Appropriate wound management for infected cord and necrotic tissue (AIII)
– Group A or B streptococci	Penicillin G IV for ≥7–14 days (shorter course for superficial funisitis without invasive infection) (AII)	Group A streptococcus usually causes "wet cord" without pus and with minimal erythema; single dose of benazthine penicillin IM adequate Consultation with pediatric ID specialist is recommended for necrotizing fasciitis (AII).
– *S aureus*	MSSA: oxacillin/nafcillin IV, IM for ≥5–7 days (shorter course for superficial funisitis without invasive infection) (AII) MRSA: vancomycin (AIII)	Assess for bacteremia and other focus of infection Alternatives for MRSA: linezolid, clindamycin (if susceptible)
– *Clostridium* spp	Clindamycin OR penicillin G IV for ≥10 days, with additional agents based on culture results (AII)	Crepitance and rapidly spreading cellulitis around umbilicus Mixed infection with other gram-positive and gram-negative bacteria common
Osteomyelitis, suppurative arthritis Obtain cultures (aerobic; fungal if NICU) of bone or joint fluid before antibiotic therapy. Duration of therapy dependent on causative organism and normalization of erythrocyte sedimentation rate and C-reactive protein; minimum for osteomyelitis 3 wk and arthritis therapy 2–3 wk if no organism identified (AIII). Surgical drainage of pus (AIII); physical therapy may be needed (BIII).		
– Empiric therapy	Nafcillin/oxacillin IV (or vancomycin if MRSA is a concern) AND cefotaxime or gentamicin IV, IM (AIII)	

Organism	Therapy	Comments
– Coliform bacteria (eg, Escherichia coli, Klebsiella sp, Enterobacter sp)	For E coli and Klebsiella: cefotaxime OR gentamicin OR ampicillin (if susceptible) (A II) For Enterobacter, Serratia, or Citrobacter: ADD gentamicin IV, IM to cefotaxime or ceftriaxone, OR use cefepime or meropenem alone (AIII)	Meropenem for ESBL-producing E coli and Klebsiella (AIII) Pip/tazo or cefepime are alternatives for susceptible bacilli (BII)
– Gonococcal arthritis and tenosynovitis	Ceftriaxone IV, IM OR cefotaxime IV x 7–10 d (AII)	Cefotaxime is preferred for infants with hyperbilirubinemia
– S aureus	MSSA: oxacillin/nafcillin IV (AII) MRSA: vancomycin IV (AIII)	Alternative for MSSA: cefazolin (AIII) Alternatives for MRSA: linezolid, clindamycin (if susceptible) (BIII), daptomycin (CIII) Addition of rifampin if persistently positive cultures
– Group B streptococcus	Ampicillin or penicillin G IV (A I)	Start with IV therapy, and switch to oral therapy when clinically stable. Amox/clav PO OR amoxicillin PO if susceptible (AIII)
– Haemophilus	Ampicillin IV, OR cefotaxime IV, IM if ampicillin-resistant	In addition to Pneumococcus and Haemophilus, coliforms and S aureus may also cause AOM in neonates (AIII)
Otitis media	No controlled treatment trials in newborns; if no response, obtain middle ear fluid for culture	
– Empiric therapy	oxacillin/nafcillin AND cefotaxime or gentamicin	Start with IV therapy, and switch to oral therapy when clinically stable Amox/clav (AIII)
– E coli (therapy of other coliforms based on susceptibility testing)	Cefotaxime OR gentamicin	Start with IV therapy, and switch to oral therapy when clinically stable Amox/clav if susceptible (AIII)
– S aureus	MSSA: oxacillin/nafcillin IV (MSSA) MRSA: vancomycin or clindamycin IV (if susceptible)	Start with IV therapy, and switch to oral therapy when clinically stable. MSSA: cephalexin PO for 10 days or cloxacillin PO (AIII) MRSA: linezolid PO or clindamycin PO (BII)
– Group A or B streptococcus	Penicillin G or ampicillin IV, IM	Start with IV therapy, and switch to oral therapy when clinically stable. Amoxicillin 30–40 mg/kg/day PO div q8h for 10 days

A. RECOMMENDED THERAPY FOR SELECTED NEWBORN CONDITIONS (cont)

Condition	Therapy (evidence grade) See Table 5B for Neonatal Dosages	Comments
Parotitis, suppurative	Oxacillin/nafcillin IV, IM for 10 days; consider vancomycin if MRSA suspected (AIII)	Usually staphylococcal but occasionally coliform Antimicrobial regimen without incision/drainage is adequate in >75% of cases.
Pulmonary infections		
- Empiric therapy of the neonate with early onset of pulmonary infiltrates (within the first 48–72 hours of life)	Ampicillin IV/IM AND gentamicin or cefotaxime IV/IM for 10 days	For newborns with no additional risk factors for bacterial infection (eg, maternal amnionitis) who have (1) negative blood cultures, (2) no need for >8 h of oxygen, and (3) are asymptomatic at 48 h into therapy, 4 days may be sufficient therapy, based on limited data.
- Aspiration pneumonia	Clindamycin IV, IM AND gentamicin IV, IM for 7–10 days (AIII)	Mild aspiration episodes may not require antibiotic therapy.
- Chlamydia trachomatis	Azithromycin PO, IV q24h for 5 days or erythromycin ethylsuccinate PO for 14 days (AII)	Association of erythromycin and pyloric stenosis in young infants
- Mycoplasma hominis	Clindamycin PO, IV for 10 days (organisms are resistant to macrolides)	Pathogenic role in pneumonia not well defined and clinical efficacy unknown; no association with bronchopulmonary dysplasia (BIII).
- Pertussis	Azithromycin 10 mg/kg PO, IV q24h for 5 days, or erythromycin ethylsuccinate PO for 14 days (AII)	Association of erythromycin and pyloric stenosis in young infants; may also occur with azithromycin Alternatives for >1 mo of age, clarithromycin for 7 days, and for >2 mo of age, TMP/SMX for 14 days
- P aeruginosa	Ceftazidime IV, IM AND tobramycin IV, IM for ≥10–14 days (AIII)	Alternatives: cefepime or meropenem, OR pip/tazo AND tobramycin

– S aureus	MSSA: oxacillin/nafcillin IV for 21 days minimum (AIII) MRSA: vancomycin IV OR clindamycin IV if susceptible (AIII) for 21 days minimum	Alternative for MSSA: cefazolin IV Addition of rifampin or linezolid if persistently positive cultures (AIII) Thoracostomy drainage of empyema
– Group B streptococcus	Penicillin G IV OR ampicillin IV, IM for 10 days (AIII)	For serious infections, ADD gentamicin for synergy until clinically improved No prospective, randomized data on the efficacy of a 7-day treatment course
– Ureaplasma spp (urealyticum or parvum)	Azithromycin PO/IV for 5 days or clarithromycin PO for 10 days (BIII)	Pathogenic role of Ureaplasma not well defined and no prophylaxis recommended for CLD Many Ureaplasma spp resistant to erythromycin Association of erythromycin and pyloric stenosis in young infants
RSV	Prevention of infection with palivizumab (Synagis) at 15 mg/kg IM, monthly during the RSV season in high-risk infants (A): 1. Infants <24 mo of age with chronic lung disease and requiring medical therapy (max 5 doses) 2. Infants <24 mo of age with hemodynamically significant congenital heart disease (max 5 doses) 3. Premature infants: (a) GA ≤28 wk, and CA <12 mo at the start of the season; (b) GA 29–<32 wk, and CA <6 mo at the start of the season; (c) GA from 32–<35 wk, and CA <3 mo before or during RSV season AND 1 of 2 risk factors (child care attendance, sibling <5 y of age) (max 3 doses) 4. Infants <35 wk GA and <12 mo of age with congenital abnormalities of airway or neuromuscular disorder	Aerosol ribavirin provides little, if any, benefit and should only be used for life-threatening infection with RSV. Difficulties in administration, complications with airway reactivity, and concern for potential toxicities to health care workers preclude routine use. Palivizumab was not investigated to treat an active infection. Palivizumab may benefit immunocompromised children and those with cystic fibrosis, but is not routinely recommended as benefits not well defined.

A. RECOMMENDED THERAPY FOR SELECTED NEWBORN CONDITIONS (cont)

Pulmonary infections (cont)

Condition	Therapy (evidence grade) See Table 5B for Neonatal Dosages	Comments
Sepsis and meningitis	*NOTE:* Duration of therapy: 10 days for sepsis without a focus (AIII); minimum of 21 days for gram-negative meningitis (or at least 14 days after CSF is sterile) and 14–21 days for GBS meningitis and other gram-positive bacteria (AIII)	There are no prospective, controlled studies on 5- or 7-day courses for mild or presumed sepsis.
– Initial therapy, organism unknown	Ampicillin IV AND cefotaxime IV (AII), OR ampicillin IV AND gentamicin IV, IM (AII)	Cefotaxime preferred if meningitis suspected or cannot be excluded (AIII) Initial empiric therapy of nosocomial infection should be based on each hospital's pathogens and susceptibilities.
– *Bacteroides fragilis*	Metronidazole or meropenem IV, IM (AIII)	Alternative; clindamycin but increasing resistance reported
– *Enterococcus* spp	Ampicillin IV, IM AND gentamicin IV, IM (AIII); for ampicillin-resistant organisms: vancomycin AND gentamicin (AIII)	Gentamicin needed with either ampicillin or vancomycin for bactericidal activity; continue until clinical and microbiological response documented (AIII) For vancomycin-resistant enterococci that are also ampicillin resistant: linezolid (AIII)
– *E coli*	Cefotaxime IV, IM or gentamicin IV, IM (AII) if no CNS infection.	Meropenem or cefepime for gentamicin/cefotaxime-resistant coliforms (eg, *Enterobacter*, *Serratia*) (AIII) Meropenem for ESBL-producing coliforms (AIII)
– Gonococcal	Ceftriaxone IV, IM OR cefotaxime IV, IM (AIII)	Duration of therapy not well defined, consider 5 days.
– *Listeria monocytogenes*	Ampicillin IV, IM AND gentamicin IV, IM (AIII)	Gentamicin is synergistic in vitro with ampicillin. Continue until clinical and microbiological response documented (AIII).

– P aeruginosa	Ceftazidime IV, IM AND tobramycin IV, IM (AIII)	Meropenem, cefepime, OR AND tobramycin are suitable alternatives (AIII). Pip/tazo should not be used for CNS infection.
– S aureus	MSSA: oxacillin/nafcillin IV, IM, or cefazolin IV, IM (AII) MRSA: vancomycin IV (AII)	Alternatives for MRSA: clindamycin, linezolid
– Staphylococcus epidermidis (or any coagulase-negative staphylococci)	Vancomycin IV (AIII)	If organism susceptible and infection not severe, oxacillin/nafcillin or cefazolin are alternatives for methicillin-susceptible strains. Cefazolin does not enter CNS. Add rifampin if cultures persistently positive. Alternative: linezolid
– Group A streptococcus	Penicillin G or ampicillin IV (AII)	
– Group B streptococcus	Ampicillin or penicillin G IV AND gentamicin IV, IM (AII)	Continue gentamicin until clinical and microbiological response documented (AIII). Duration of therapy: 10 days for bacteremia/sepsis (AII); minimum of 14 days for meningitis (AII)
Skin and soft tissues		
– Breast abscess	Vancomycin IV (for MRSA) or oxacillin/nafcillin IV, IM (MSSA) AND cefotaxime OR gentamicin if gram-negative rods seen on Gram stain (AII)	Gram stain of expressed pus guides empiric therapy; vancomycin if MRSA prevalent in community; alternative to vancomycin: clindamycin, linezolid, may need surgical drainage to minimize damage to breast tissue Treatment duration individualized, until clinical findings have completely resolved (AIII)
– Erysipelas (and other group A streptococcal infections)	Penicillin G IV for 5–7 days, followed by oral therapy (if bacteremia not present) to complete a 10-day course (AIII)	Alternative: ampicillin GBS may produce similar cellulitis or nodular lesions.

A. RECOMMENDED THERAPY FOR SELECTED NEWBORN CONDITIONS (cont)

Condition	Therapy (evidence grade) See Table 5B for Neonatal Dosages	Comments
Skin and soft tissues (cont)		
– Impetigo neonatorum	MSSA: oxacillin/nafcillin IV, IM OR cephalexin (AIII) MRSA: vancomycin IV; for 5 days (AIII)	Systemic antibiotic therapy usually not required for superficial impetigo; local chlorhexidine cleansing may help with or without topical mupirocin (MRSA) or bacitracin (MSSA). Alternatives for MRSA: clindamycin IV, PO, or linezolid IV, PO
– S aureus	MSSA: oxacillin/nafcillin IV, IM (AII) MRSA: vancomycin IV (AIII)	Surgical drainage may be required. MRSA may cause necrotizing fasciitis. Alternatives for MRSA: clindamycin IV or linezolid IV Convalescent oral therapy if infection responds quickly to IV therapy
– Group B streptococcus	Penicillin G IV OR ampicillin IV, IM	Usually no pus formed Treatment course dependent on extent of infection, 7–14 days
Syphilis, congenital (AIII) (<1 mo of age)	During periods when the availability of penicillin is compromised, see http://www.cdc.gov/nchstp/dstd/penicillinG.htm.	Evaluation and treatment do not depend on mother's HIV status. Obtain follow-up serology every 2–3 mo until nontreponemal test nonreactive or decreased 4-fold. If CSF positive, repeat spinal tap with CSF VDRL at 6 mo, and if abnormal, re-treat.

– Proven or highly probable disease: (1) abnormal physical exam; (2) serum quantitative nontreponemal serologic titer that is 4-fold higher than the mother's titer; or (3) a positive darkfield or fluorescent antibody test of body fluid(s)	Aqueous penicillin G 50,000 U/kg/dose q12h (day of life 1–7), q8h (>7 days) IV OR procaine penicillin G 50,000 U/kg IM q24h; for 10 days (All)	Evaluation to determine type and duration of therapy: CSF analysis (VDRL, cell count, protein), CBC and platelet count. Other tests as clinically indicated, including long-bone radiographs, chest radiograph, liver function tests, cranial ultrasound, ophthalmologic exam, and hearing test (auditory brainstem response) If >1 day of therapy is missed, the entire course is restarted.
– Normal physical exam, serum quantitative nontreponemal serologic titer ≤ maternal titer and maternal treatment was (1) none, inadequate, or undocumented; (2) erythromycin, azithromycin, or other non-penicillin regimen; or (3) <4 wk before delivery	Evaluation abnormal or not done completely: aqueous penicillin G 50,000 U/kg/dose q12h (day of life 1–7), q8h (>7 days) IV OR procaine penicillin G 50,000 U/kg IM q24h for 10 days (All) Evaluation normal: aqueous penicillin G 50,000 U/kg/dose q12h (day of life 1–7), q8h (>7 days) IV OR procaine penicillin G 50,000 U/kg IM q24h for 10 days; OR benzathine penicillin G 50,000 units/kg/dose IM in a single dose	Evaluation: CSF analysis, CBC with platelets, long-bone radiographs If >1 day of therapy is missed, the entire course is restarted. Reliable follow-up important if only a single dose of benzathine penicillin given.
– Normal physical exam, serum quantitative nontreponemal serologic titer ≤ maternal titer; mother treated adequately during pregnancy and >4 wk before delivery; no evidence of reinfection or relapse in mother	Benzathine penicillin G 50,000 units/kg/dose IM in a single dose (All)	No evaluation required. Some experts would not treat but provide close serologic follow-up.

A. RECOMMENDED THERAPY FOR SELECTED NEWBORN CONDITIONS (cont)

Condition	Therapy (evidence grade) See Table 5B for Neonatal Dosages	Comments
– Normal physical exam, serum quantitative nontreponemal serologic titer ≤ maternal titer, and the mother's treatment was adequate before pregnancy	No treatment	No evaluation required. Some experts would treat with benzathine penicillin G 50,000 units/kg as a single IM injection, particularly if follow-up is uncertain.
Syphilis, congenital (>1 mo of age)	Aqueous crystalline penicillin G 200,000–300,000 units/kg/day IV div q4–6h for 10 days (AII)	Evaluation to determine type and duration of therapy: CSF analysis (VDRL, cell count, protein), CBC and platelet count. Other tests as clinically indicated, including long-bone radiographs, chest radiograph, liver function tests, neuroimaging, ophthalmologic exam, and hearing evaluation. If no clinical manifestations of disease, the CSF exam is normal, and the CSF VDRL test result is nonreactive, some specialists would treat with up to 3 weekly doses of benzathine penicillin G, 50,000 U/kg IM. Some experts would provide a single dose of benzathine penicillin G, 50,000 U/kg IM after the 10 days of parenteral treatment, but the value of this additional therapy is not well documented.
Tetanus neonatorum	Metronidazole IV/PO (alternative: penicillin G IV for 10–14 days (AIII) Human TIG 3,000–6,000 U IM for 1 dose (AIII)	Wound cleaning and debridement vital; IVIG (200–400 mg/kg) is an alternative if TIG not available; equine tetanus antitoxin not available in US but is alternative to TIG
Toxoplasmosis, congenital	Sulfadiazine 100 mg/kg/day PO div q12h AND pyrimethamine 2 mg/kg PO daily for 2 days (loading dose), then 1 mg/kg PO q24h for 2–6 mo, then 3 times weekly (M-W-F) up to 1 y (AII) Folinic acid (leukovorin) 10 mg 3 times weekly (AII)	Corticosteroids (1 mg/kg/day div q12h) if active chorioretinitis or CSF protein >1 g/dL (AIII) Start sulfa after neonatal jaundice has resolved. Therapy is only effective against active trophozoites, not cysts.

Urinary tract infection	Initial empiric therapy with ampicillin AND gentamicin; OR ampicillin AND cefotaxime pending culture and susceptibility test results for 7–10 days	Investigate for kidney disease and for abnormalities of urinary tract: VCUG indicated if renal ultrasound abnormal or after 1st UTI Oral therapy acceptable once infant asymptomatic and culture sterile. No prophylaxis for Grades 1–3 reflux.
– Coliform bacteria (eg, E coli, Klebsiella, Enterobacter, Serratia)	Cefotaxime IV, IM OR, in the absence of renal or perinephric abscess, gentamicin IV, IM for 7–10 days (AII)	Ampicillin used for susceptible organisms
– Enterococcus	Ampicillin IV, IM for 7 days for cystitis, may need 10–14 days for pyelonephritis, add gentamicin until cultures are sterile (AII); for ampicillin resistance, use vancomycin, add gentamicin until cultures are sterile	Aminoglycoside needed with ampicillin or vancomycin for bactericidal activity (assuming organisms susceptible to an aminoglycoside)
– P aeruginosa	Ceftazidime IV, IM OR, in the absence of renal or perinephric abscess, tobramycin IV, IM for 7–10 days (AIII)	Meropenem or cefepime are alternatives.
– Candida spp	AmB-D IV OR fluconazole (if susceptible) (AII)	Evaluate for other sites in high-risk neonates: CSF analysis; cardiac ECHO; abdominal ultrasound to include kidneys, bladder; eye exam. Other triazoles are alternatives; insufficient data on echinocandins for neonatal UTI.

B. ANTIMICROBIAL DOSAGES FOR NEONATES

		Dosages (mg/kg/day) and Intervals of Administration				
		Chronologic Age ≤28 days				Chronologic Age >28 days
		Body Weight ≤2,000 g		Body Weight >2,000 g		
Antibiotic	Route	0–7 days old	8–28 days old	0–7 days old	8–28 days old	Chronologic Age >28 days
Acyclovir	IV	40 div q12h	60 div q8h	60 div q8h	60 div q8h	60 div q8h
Amoxicillin/clavulanate	PO			30 div q12h	30 div q12h	30 div q12h
Amphotericin B						
– deoxycholate	IV	1 q24h	1 q24h	1 q24h	1 q24h	1 q24h
– lipid complex	IV	5 q24h	5 q24h	5 q24h	5 q24h	5 q24h
– liposomal	IV	5 q24h	5 q24h	5 q24h	5 q24h	5 q24h
Ampicillin	IV, IM	100 div q12h	150 div q8h	150 div q8h	200 div q6h	200 div q6h
Anidulafungin	IV	1.5 q24	1.5 q24	1.5 q24	1.5 q24	1.5 q24
Azithromycin	PO	10 q24h	10 q24h	10 q24h	10 q24h	10 q24h
	IV	10 q24h	10 q24h	10 q24h	10 q24h	10 q24h
Aztreonam	IV, IM	60 div q12h	90 div q8h	60 div q12h	90 div q8h	120 div q6h
Caspofungin	IV	25/m² q24h	25/m² q24h	25/m² q24h	25/m² q24h	25/m² q24h
Cefazolin	IV, IM	50 div q12h	50 div q12h	50 div q12h	75 div q8h	75 div q8h
Cefepime	IV, IM	100 div q12h	150 div q8h	150 div q8h	150 div q8h	150 div q8h
Cefotaxime	IV, IM	100 div q12h	150 div q8h	100 div q12h	150 div q8h	200 div q6h
Ceftazidime	IV, IM	100 div q12h	150 div q8h	100 div q12h	150 div q8h	150 div q8h
Ceftriaxone	IV, IM	50 q24h	50 q24h	50 q24h	50 q24h	50 q24h
Cefuroxime	IV, IM	100 div q12h	150 div q8h	100 div q12h	150 div q8h	150 div q8h

Drug	Route						
Chloramphenicol	IV, IM	25 q24h	50 div q12h	25 q24h	25 q24h	50 div q12h	50-100 div q6h
Clindamycin	IV, IM, PO	10 div q12h	15 div q8h	15 div q8h	15 div q8h	20 div q6h	30 div q6h
Daptomycin	IV	12 div q12h	12 div q12h	12 div q12h	12 div q12h	12 div q12h	12 div q12h
Erythromycin	PO	20 div q12h	30 div q8h	20 div q12h	20 div q12h	30 div q8h	40 div q6h
Fluconazole							
– treatment	IV, PO	12 q24h	12 q24h	12 q24h	12 q24h	12 q24h	12 q24h
– prophylaxis	IV, PO	3 twice wkly	3 twice wkly	3 twice wkly	3 twice wkly	3 twice wkly	3 twice wkly
Flucytosine	PO	75 div q8h	75 div q6h	75 div q6h	75 div q6h	75 div q6h	75 div q6h
Ganciclovir	IV	See text: CMV	See text: CMV	12 div q12h	12 div q12h	12 div q12h	12 div q12h
Linezolid	IV, PO	20 div q12h	30 div q8h	30 div q8h	30 div q8h	30 div q8h	30 div q8h
Meropenem							
– sepsis	IV	40 div q12h	60 div q8h	60 div q8h	60 div q8h	90 div q8h	90 div q8h
– meningitis	IV	120 div q8h	120 div q8h	120 civ q8h	120 div q8h	120 div q8h	120 div q8h
Metronidazole	IV, PO	7.5 q24-48h	15 c24h	15 q24h	30 div q12h	30 div q12h	30 div q8h
Micafungin	IV	10 q24h	10 c24h	10 q24h	10 q24h	10 q24h	10 q24h
Nafcillin, oxacillin	IV, IM	50 div q12h	75 div q8h	75 div q8h	75 div q8h	100 div q6h	150 div q6h
Penicillin G benzathine	IM	50,000 U	50,000 U	50,000 U	50,000 U	50,000 U	50,000 U
Penicillin G crystalline (CBS meningitis)	IV	200,000 U div q12h	300,000 U div q8h	300,000 U div q8h	300,000 U div q6h	400,000 U div q6h	400,000 U div q6h
Penicillin G crystalline (congenital syphilis)	IV	100,000 U div q12h	150,000 U div q8h	100,000 U div q12h	100,000 U div q12h	150,000 U div q8h	200,000 U div q6h
Penicillin G procaine	IM	50,000 U q24h	50,000 U q24h	50,000 U q24h	50,000 U q24h	50,000 U q24h	50,000 U q24h

B. ANTIMICROBIAL DOSAGES FOR NEONATES (cont)

		Dosages (mg/kg/day) and Intervals of Administration				
		Chronologic Age ≤28 days				Chronologic Age >28 days
		Body Weight ≤2,000 g		Body Weight >2,000 g		
Antibiotic	Route	0–7 days old	8–28 days old	0–7 days old	8–28 days old	
Piperacillin/tazobactam	IV	200 div q12h	300 div q8h	200 div q12h	300 div q8h	400 div q6h
Rifampin	IV, PO	10 q24h	10 q24h	10 q24h	10 q24h	10 q24h
Ticarcillin/clavulanate	IV	150 div q12h	225 div q8h	150 div 12h	225 div q8h	300 div q6h
Valganciclovir	PO	See text: CMV	See text: CMV	32 div q12h	32 div q12h	32 div q12h
Voriconazole	IV, PO	8–16 div q12h	8–16 div q12h	8–16 div q12h	8–16 div q12h	8–16 div q12h
Zidovudine	IV	3 div q12h	3 div q12h	6 div q6h	6 div q6h	See text: HIV
	PO	4 div12h	4 div q12h	8 div q12h	8 div q12h	See text: HIV

C. AMINOGLYCOSIDES

Medication	Route	Empiric Dosage (mg/kg/DOSE) by Gestational and Postnatal Age					
		<32 wk		32–36 wk		≥37 wk (term)	
		0–14 days	>14 days	0–7 days	>7 days	0–7 days	>7 days
Amikacin	IV, IM	15 q48	15 q24	15 q24	15 q24h	15 q24h	15 q24
Gentamicin	IV, IM	5 q48h	5 q36h	4 q36h	4 q24h	4 q24h	4 q24h
Tobramycin	IV, IM	5 q48h	5 q36h	4 q36h	4 q24h	4 q24h	4 q24h

D. VANCOMYCIN

Empiric Dosage (mg/kg/DOSE) by Gestational Age and Serum Creatinine					
≤28 wk			>28 wk		
Serum Creatinine	Dose	Frequency	Serum Creatinine	Dose	Frequency
<0.5	15	q12h	<0.7	15	q12h
0.5–0.7	20	q24h	0.7–0.9	20	q24h
0.8–1	15	q24h	1–1.2	15	q24h
1.1–1.4	10	q24h	1.3–1.6	10	q24h
>1.4	15	q48h	>1.6	15	q48h

E. Use of Antimicrobials During Pregnancy or Breastfeeding

The use of antimicrobials during pregnancy should be balanced by the risk of fetal toxicity, including anatomical anomalies. A number of factors determine the degree of transfer of antibiotics across the placenta: lipid solubility, degree of ionization, molecular weight, protein binding, placental maturation, and placental and fetal blood flow. The FDA provides 5 categories to indicate the level of risk to the fetus: (1) Category A: fetal harm seems remote since controlled studies have not demonstrated a risk to the fetus; (2) Category B: animal reproduction studies have not shown a fetal risk but no controlled studies in pregnant women have been done, or animal studies have shown an adverse effect that has not been confirmed in human studies (penicillin, amoxicillin, ampicillin, cephalexin/cefazolin, azithromycin, clindamycin, vancomycin, zanamivir); (3) Category C: studies in animals have shown an adverse effect on the fetus but there are no studies in women and no animal data are available; the potential benefit of the drug may justify the possible risk to the fetus (chloramphenicol, ciprofloxacin, gentamicin, levofloxacin, oseltamivir, rifampin); (4) Category D: evidence exists of human fetal risk but the benefits may outweigh such risk (doxycycline); (5) Category X: The drug is contraindicated since animal or human studies have shown fetal abnormalities or fetal risk (ribavirin).

The most current, updated information can be found at the National Library of Medicine Web site (http://www.toxnet.nlm.nih.gov/cgi-bin/sis/htmlgen?LACT). This Web site provides the Drugs and Lactation Database (LactMed), which contains a peer-reviewed and fully referenced database of drugs to which breastfeeding mothers may be exposed. Among the data included are maternal and infant levels of drugs, possible effects on breastfed infants and on lactation, and alternate drugs to consider. Just type in the drug for which you need information, and the full report on that drug is provided.

Fetal serum concentrations of the following commonly used drugs are equal to, or only slightly less than, those in the mother: penicillin G, amoxicillin, ampicillin, sulfonamides, trimethoprim, tetracyclines, and nitrofurantoin. The aminoglycoside concentrations in fetal serum are 20% to 50% of those in maternal serum. Cephalosporins, nafcillin, oxacillin, and clindamycin penetrate poorly (10%–15%), and fetal concentrations of erythromycin and dicloxacillin are less than 10% of those in the mother.

The use of antimicrobials by the mother during breastfeeding should be balanced by the risk of clinical or laboratory toxicities in the infant. In general, the neonatal exposure is well tolerated. While maternal treatment with sulfa-containing antibiotics should be approached with caution in the breastfed infant who is jaundiced or ill, no neonatal symptoms have been associated with maternal treatment with amoxicillin, cefazolin, cefotaxime, ceftazidime, ceftriaxone, ciprofloxacin, clindamycin, erythromycin, ethambutol, fluconazole, gentamicin, isoniazid, and rifampin (used for <3 weeks). Metronidazole seems safe, but may impart a metallic taste to breast milk.

6. Antimicrobial Therapy According to Clinical Syndromes

NOTES

- This chapter should be considered a rough guideline for a typical patient. Dosage recommendations are for patients with relatively normal hydration, renal function, and hepatic function. See Chapter 13 for information on patients with impaired renal function. Higher dosages may be necessary if the antibiotic does not penetrate well into the infected tissue (eg, meningitis), or if the child is immunocompromised.

- Duration of treatment should be individualized. Those recommended are based on the literature, common practice, and general experience. Critical evaluations of duration of therapy have been carried out in very few infectious diseases. In general, a longer duration of therapy should be used (1) for tissues in which antibiotic concentrations may be relatively low (eg, abscess, CNS infection) and tissues in which repair following infection-mediated damage is slow (eg, bone), (2) when the organisms are less susceptible, (3) when a relapse of infection is unacceptable (eg, CNS infections), or (4) when the host is immunocompromised in some way. An assessment after therapy will ensure that your selection of antibiotic, dose, and duration of therapy was appropriate.

- Diseases are arranged by body systems. Consult the index for the alphabetized listing of diseases and Chapters 7 through 10 for the alphabetized listing of pathogens and for uncommon organisms not included in this chapter.

- **Abbreviations:** ADH, antidiuretic hormone; AFB, acid-fast bacilli; amox/clav, amoxicillin/clavulanate; amp/sulbactam, ampicillin/sulbactam; AOM, acute otitis media; bid, twice daily; CA-MRSA, community-associated methicillin-resistant *Staphylococcus aureus*; CDC, Centers for Disease Control and Prevention; CMV, cytomegalovirus; CNS, central nervous system; CSF, cerebrospinal fluid; CT, computed tomography; div, divided; EBV, Epstein-Barr virus; ESBL, extended spectrum beta-lactamase; ESR, erythrocyte sedimentation rate; FDA, US Food and Drug Administration; GI, gastrointestinal; HIV, human immunodeficiency virus; HSV, herpes simplex virus; HUS, hemolytic uremic syndrome; I&D, incision and drainage; IDSA, Infectious Diseases Society of America; IM, intramuscular; INH, isoniazid; IV, intravenous; IVIG, intravenous immune globulin; LP, lumbar puncture; MRSE, methicillin-resistant *Staphylococcus epidermidis*; MSSA, methicillin-susceptible *S aureus*; MSSE, methicillin-sensitive *S epidermidis*; NIH, National Institutes of Health; ophth, ophthalmic; PCV7, Prevnar 7-valent pneumococcal conjugate vaccine; PCV13, Prevnar 13-valent pneumococcal conjugate vaccine; pen-R, penicillin-resistant; pen-S, penicillin-susceptible; pip/tazo, piperacillin/tazobactam; PO, oral; PPD, purified protein derivative; PZA, pyrazinamide; qd, once daily; qid, 4 times daily; qod, every other day; RSV, respiratory syncytial virus; SPAG-2, small particle aerosol generator-2; STI, sexually transmitted infection; soln, solution; ticar/clav, ticarcillin/clavulanate; tid, 3 times daily; TB, tuberculosis; TMP/SMX, trimethoprim/sulfamethoxazole; USP-NF, US Pharmacopeia–National Formulary; UTI, urinary tract infection; VDRL, Venereal Disease Research Laboratories; WBC, white blood cell.

A. SKIN AND SOFT TISSUE INFECTIONS

Clinical Diagnosis	Therapy (evidence grade)	Comments
NOTE: CA-MRSA (see Chapter 4 on CA-MRSA) is increasingly prevalent in most areas of the world. Recommendations below are given for 2 scenarios, "CA-MRSA" and "standard." Antibiotic recommendations for CA-MRSA should be used for empiric therapy when CA-MRSA is suspected and for documented CA-MRSA infections, while "standard" recommendations refer to treatment of MSSA. Please check your local susceptibility data for *S aureus* before using clindamycin for empiric therapy. For MSSA, oxacillin/nafcillin are considered equivalent agents.		
Adenitis, acute bacterial (*S aureus*, including CA-MRSA, and group A streptococcus)	Empiric IV therapy: Standard: oxacillin/nafcillin 150 mg/kg/day IV div q6h OR cefazolin 100 mg/kg/day IV div q8h (AI) CA-MRSA: clindamycin 30 mg/kg/day IV div q8h OR vancomycin 40 mg/kg/day IV q8h (BII)	May need surgical drainage For oral therapy for MSSA: cephalexin OR cloxacillin; for CA-MRSA: clindamycin, TMP/SMX, or linezolid For group A strep: amoxicillin Total PO therapy for 7–10 days
Adenitis, nontuberculous (atypical) mycobacterial	Excision usually curative (BII); azithromycin PO OR clarithromycin PO for 6–12 wk (with or without rifampin) if susceptible (BII)	Antibiotic susceptibility patterns are quite variable; cultures should guide therapy; medical therapy 60%–70% effective. Newer data suggest toxicity of anti-microbials may not be worth the small clinical benefit.
Adenitis, tuberculous	Isoniazid 10–15 mg/kg/day (max 300 mg) PO qd AND rifampin 10–20 mg/kg/day (max 600 mg) PO qd, IV for 6 mo AND PZA 20–40 mg/kg/day PO qd for first 2 mo therapy (BI); if suspected multidrug resistance, add ethambutol 20 mg/kg/day PO qd	Surgical excision usually not indicated Adenitis caused by *Mycobacterium bovis* (unpasteurized dairy product ingestion) is uniformly resistant to PZA. Treat 9–12 mo with isoniazid and rifampin, if susceptible (BII).
Anthrax, cutaneous	Empiric therapy: ciprofloxacin 20–30 mg/kg/day PO bid OR doxycycline 4 mg/kg/day PO bid (max 200 mg) PO div bid (regardless of age) (AIII)	If susceptible, amoxicillin or clindamycin (BII). Ciprofloxacin and levofloxacin are FDA approved for inhalation anthrax (BII).
Bites, animal and human *Pasteurella multocida* (animal), *Eikenella corrodens* (human), *Staphylococcus* species and *Streptococcus* species	Amox/clav 45 mg/kg/day PO tid (amox/clav 7:1, see Chapter 1, Aminopenicillins) for 5–10 days (AII); for hospitalized children, use ticar/clav 200 mg ticarcillin/kg/day div q6h OR ampicillin and clindamycin (BII)	Consider rabies prophylaxis for animal bites (AI); consider tetanus prophylaxis. Human bites have a very high rate of infection (do not close open wounds). *S aureus* coverage is only fair with amox/clav, ticar/clav, pip/tazo. For penicillin allergy, consider ciprofloxacin (for *Pasteurella*) plus clindamycin (BIII).

Infection	Therapy	Comments
Bullous impetigo (usually *S aureus*, including CA-MRSA)	Standard: cephalexin 50–75 mg/kg/day PO div tid OR amox/clav 45 mg/kg/day PO div tid (CII) CA-MRSA: clindamycin 30 mg/kg/day PO div tid OR TMP/SMX 8 mg/kg/day of TMP PO div bid; for 5–7 days (CIII)	For topical therapy if mild infection: mupirocin or retapamulin ointment
Cellulitis of unknown etiology (usually *S aureus*, including CA-MRSA, or group A streptococcus)	Empiric IV therapy: Standard: oxacillin/nafcillin 150 mg/kg/day IV div q6h OR cefazolin 100 mg/kg/day IV c iv q8h (BII) CA-MRSA: clindamycin 30 mg/kg/day IV div q8h OR vancomycin 40 mg/kg/day IV q8h (BII) For oral therapy for MSSA: cephalexin (AII) OR amox/clav 45 mg/kg/day PO d v tid (3II); for CA-MRSA: clindamycin (BII), TMP/SMX (CIII), or linezolid. (BII)	For periorbital or buccal cellulitis also consider *Streptococcus pneumoniae* or *Haemophilus influenzae* type b in unimmunized infants Total IV plus PO therapy for 7–10 days
Cellulitis, buccal (*H influenzae*, type b)	Cefotaxime 100–150 mg/day IV div q8h OR ceftriaxone 50 mg/kg/day (AII) IV, IM q24h; for 2–7 days parenteral therapy before switch to oral (BII)	Rule out meningitis (larger dosages may be needed). For penicillin allergy, levofloxacin IV/PO covers pathogens, but no clinical data available; safer than chloramphenicol. Oral therapy: amoxicillin if beta-lactamase negative; amox/clav or oral 2nd or 3rd generation cephalosporin if beta-lactamase positive
Cellulitis, erysipelas (streptococcal)	Penicillin G 100,000–200,000 U/kg/day IV div q4–6h (BII) initially then penicillin V 100 mg/kg/day PO div qid or tid OR amoxicillin 50 mg/kg/day PO div tid for 10 days	These dosages may be unnecessarily large, but there is little clinical experience with smaller dosages.
Gas gangrene (clostridial)	Penicillin G 250,000 U/kg/day IV div q4h (BII) for 10 days; for penicillin allergy; clindamycin or meropenem (CIII)	Aggressive, extensive debridement

A. SKIN AND SOFT TISSUE INFECTIONS (cont)

Clinical Diagnosis	Therapy (evidence grade)	Comments
Impetigo (S aureus, including CA-MRSA; occasionally group A streptococcus)	Mupirocin OR retapamulin topically (BII) to lesions tid; OR for more extensive lesions, oral therapy: Standard: cephalexin 50–75 mg/kg/day PO div tid OR amox/clav 45 mg/kg/day PO div tid (AII) CA-MRSA: clindamycin 30 mg/kg/day PO div tid OR TMP/SMX 8 mg/kg/day of TMP PO div bid (CIII); for 5–7 days	Cleanse infected area with soap and water; bathe daily.
Ludwig angina	Penicillin G 200,000–250,000 U/kg/day IV div q6h AND clindamycin 40 mg/kg/day IV div q8h (CIII)	Alternatives: meropenem, imipenem, ticar/clav, pip/tazo if gram-negative aerobic bacilli also suspected (CIII); high risk of respiratory tract obstruction from inflammatory edema
Lymphadenitis (see Adenitis, acute bacterial)		
Lymphangitis, blistering dactylitis (group A streptococcus)	Penicillin G 200,000 U/kg/day IV div q6h (BII) initially then penicillin V 100 mg/kg/day PO div qid OR amoxicillin 50 mg/kg/day PO div tid for 10 days	For mild disease, penicillin V 50 mg/kg/day PO div qid OR erythromycin 40 mg/kg/day PO div tid for 10 days
Myositis, suppurative (S aureus, including CA-MRSA; synonyms: tropical myositis, pyomyositis)	Standard: oxacillin/nafcillin 150 mg/kg/day IV div q6h OR cefazolin 100 mg/kg/day IV div q8h (CII) CA-MRSA: clindamycin 40 mg/kg/day IV div q8h OR vancomycin 40 mg/kg/day IV div q8h (CIII)	Aggressive, emergent debridement; consider IVIG to bind bacterial toxins for life-threatening disease; use clindamycin to help decrease toxin production; abscesses may develop with CA-MRSA while on therapy.

Necrotizing fasciitis (pathogens vary, depending on the age of the child and location of infection: Single pathogen: group A streptococcus; *Clostridia* spp, *S aureus* [including CA-MRSA], *Pseudomonas aeruginosa*, *Vibrio* spp, *Aeromonas*; multiple pathogen, mixed aerobic/anaerobic synergistic fasciitis: any organism[s] above, plus gram-negative bacilli, plus *Bacteroides* spp, and other anaerobes)	Empiric therapy: ceftazidime 150 mg/kg/day IV div q8h, or cefepime 150 mg/kg/day IV div q6h or cefotaxime 200 mg/kg/day IV div q6h AND clindamycin 40 mg/kg/day IV div q6h (BIII); OR meropenem 60 mg/kg/day IV div q8h; OR pip/tazo 400 mg/kg/day pip component IV div q6h (AII) ADD vancomycin for suspect CA-MRSA, pending culture results (AIII) Group A streptococcal: penicillin G 200,000–250,000 U/kg/day div q6h AND clindamycin 40 mg/kg/day div q8h (AIII) Mixed aerobic/anaerobic/gram-negative: meropenem or pip/tazo AND clindamycin (AIII)	Aggressive emergent wound debridement (AII) Add clindamycin to inhibit synthesis of toxins at the ribosomal level (AIII). If CA-MRSA identified, and susceptible to clindamycin, additional vancomycin is not required. Consider IVIG to bind bacterial toxins for life-threatening disease (BIII). Value of hyperbaric oxygen is not established (CIII). Focus definitive antimicrobial therapy based on culture results.
Pyoderma, cutaneous abscesses (*S aureus*, including CA-MRSA; group A streptococcus)	Standard: cephalexin 50–75 mg/kg/day PO div tid OR amox/clav 45 mg/kg/day PO div tid (BII) CA-MRSA: clindamycin 30 mg/kg/day PO div tid (BII) OR TMP/SMX 8 mg/kg/day of TMP PO div bid (C II)	I&D when indicated; IV for serious infections. For prevention of recurrent CA-MRSA infection, use bleach baths daily (1/2 cup of bleach per full bathtub) (BII), OR bathe with chlorhexidine soap daily, or qod. Decolonization with mupirocin may also be helpful.
Rat-bite fever (*Streptobacillus moniliformis*, *Spirillum minus*)	Penicillin G 100,000–200,000 U/kg/day IV div q6h (BIII) for 7–10 days; for endocarditis, ADD gentamicin for 4–6 wk (CII); For mild disease, oral therapy with amox/clav (CIII)	Organisms are normal oral flora for rodents. High rate of associated endocarditis. Alternatives: doxycycline; 2nd and 3rd generation cephalosporins (CII)
Staphylococcal scalded skin syndrome	Standard: oxacillin 150 mg/kg/day IV div q6h OR cefazolin 100 mg/kg/day IV div q8h (CII) CA-MRSA: clindamycin 30 mg/kg/day IV div q8h (CIII) or vancomycin 40 mg/kg/day IV div q8h (CIII)	Burow or Zephiran compresses for oozing skin and intertriginous areas. Corticosteroids are contraindicated.

B. SKELETAL INFECTIONS

Clinical Diagnosis	Therapy (evidence grade)	Comments
NOTE: CA-MRSA (see Chapter 4 on CA-MRSA) is increasingly prevalent in most areas of the world. Recommendations below are given for CA-MRSA and MSSA. Antibiotic recommendations for empiric therapy should include CA-MRSA when it is suspected or documented, while treatment for MSSA with beta-lactam antibiotics (like cephalexin) is preferred over clindamycin. During the past 2 years, clindamycin resistance in MRSA has increased to 40% in some areas, but remained stable at 5% in others. Please check your local susceptibility data for *S aureus* before using clindamycin for empiric therapy. For MSSA, oxacillin/nafcillin are considered equivalent agents.		
Arthritis, bacterial	Switch to appropriate high-dose oral therapy when clinically improved (see Chapter 15).	
– Newborns	See Chapter 5.	
– Infants (*S aureus*, including CA-MRSA; group A streptococcus; *Kingella kingae*; in unimmunized or immunocompromised children: pneumococcus, *H influenzae* type b)	Empiric therapy: clindamycin (to cover CA-MRSA unless clindamycin resistance locally is >10%, then use vancomycin) For serious infections, ADD cefazolin to provide better MSSA coverage and add *Kingella* coverage For CA-MRSA: clindamycin 30 mg/kg/day IV div q8h OR vancomycin 40 mg/kg/day IV q8h For MSSA: oxacillin/nafcillin 150 mg/kg/day IV div q6h OR cefazolin 100 mg/kg/day IV div q8h For *Kingella*: cefazolin 100 mg/kg/day IV div q8h OR ampicillin 150 mg/kg/day IV div q6h, OR ceftriaxone 50 mg/kg/day IV, IM q24h	Oral therapy options: For CA-MRSA: clindamycin OR linezolid For MSSA: cephalexin OR dicloxacillin caps for older children For *Kingella*, most penicillins or cephalosporins (but not clindamycin) Total therapy (IV plus PO) for 3 wk with normal ESR; low-risk, non-hip arthritis may respond to a 10-day course.
– Children (*S aureus*, including CA-MRSA; group A streptococcus)	For pen-S pneumococci or group A streptococcus: penicillin G 200,000 U/kg/day IV div q6h For pen-R pneumococci or *Haemophilus*: ceftriaxone 50–75 mg/kg/day IV, IM q24h, OR cefotaxime (BII)	
– Gonococcal arthritis or tenosynovitis	Ceftriaxone 50 mg/kg IV, IM q24h (BII); for 7 days	PO cefixime 8 mg/kg/day as a single daily dose has not yet been studied in children, but is recommended as step-down therapy in adults, to complete a 7-day treatment course.
– Other bacteria	See Chapter 7 for preferred antibiotics.	

Osteomyelitis	Step-down to appropriate high-dose oral therapy when clinically improved (See Chapter 15.)	
– Newborn	See Chapter 5.	
– Infants and children, acute infection (usually S aureus, including CA-MRSA; group A streptococcus; K kingae)	Empiric therapy: clindamycin. For serious infections, ADD cefazolin to provide better MSSA coverage and add Kingella coverage (CIII). For CA-MRSA: clindamycin 30 mg/kg/day IV div q8h or vancomycin 40 mg/kg/day IV q6h For MSSA: oxacillin/nafcillin 150 mg/kg/day IV div q6h OR cefazolin 100 mg/kg/day IV div q8h (AII) For Kingella: cefazolin 100 mg/kg/day IV div q8h OR ampicillin 150 mg/kg/day IV div q6h, OR ceftriaxone 50 mg/kg/day IV, IM q24h (BIII) Total therapy (IV plus PO) usually 4–6 wk (with end-of-therapy normal ESR, x-ray to document healing) for MSSA. May need longer for CA-MRSA (BII). Follow closely for clinical response to empiric therapy.	In children with open fractures secondary to trauma, add ceftazidime for extended aerobic gram-negative activity. Kingella is often resistant to clindamycin. For MSSA (BI) and Kingella (BIII), step-down oral therapy with cephalexin 100 mg/kg/day PO tid. Oral step-down therapy alternatives for CA-MRSA include clindamycin and linezolid.
– Acute, other organisms	See Chapter 7 for preferred antibiotics.	
– Chronic (staphylococcal)	For MSSA: cephalexin 100 mg/kg/day PO div tid OR dicloxacillin caps 75–100 mg/kg/day PO div qid for 3–6 mo or longer (CIII) For CA-MRSA: clindamycin or linezolid (CIII)	Surgery to debride sequestrum is usually required for cure. For prosthetic joint infection caused by staphylococci, add rifampin (CIII). Watch for beta-lactam–associated neutropenia with high-dose, long-term therapy, and linezolid-associated neutropenia/thrombocytopenia with long-term (>2 wk) therapy.
Osteomyelitis of the foot (osteochondritis after a puncture wound) P aeruginosa (occasionally S aureus, including CA-MRSA)	Ceftazidime 150 mg/kg/day IV, IM div q8h AND tobramycin 6–7.5 mg/kg/day IM, IV div q8h (BIII); OR cefepime 150 mg/kg/day IV div q8h (BIII); OR meropenem 60 mg/kg/day IV div q8h (BIII); ADD vancomycin 40 mg/kg/day IV q8h for serious infection (for CA-MRSA), per ding culture results	Thorough surgical debridement required (2nd drainage procedure needed in at least 20% of children); oral convalescent therapy with ciprofloxacin (BIII) Treatment course 7–10 days after surgery

C. EYE INFECTIONS

Clinical Diagnosis	Therapy (evidence grade)	Comments
Cellulitis, orbital (usually secondary to sinus infection; caused by respiratory tract flora and S aureus, including CA-MRSA)	Cefotaxime 150 mg/kg/day div q8h or ceftriaxone 50 mg/kg/day q24h; ADD (for S aureus, including CA-MRSA): clindamycin 30 mg/kg/day IV q8h OR vancomycin 40 mg/kg/day IV q8h (AIII). If MSSA isolated, use: oxacillin/nafcillin IV OR cefazolin IV	Surgical drainage of larger collections of pus, if present by CT scan in orbit or subperiosteal tissue. Try medical therapy alone for small abscess (BIII). Treatment course for 10–14 days after surgical drainage, up to 21 days. CT scan to confirm cure (BIII).
Cellulitis, periorbital (preseptal infection)		
– Associated with entry site lesion on skin (S aureus, including CA-MRSA, group A streptococcus)	Standard: oxacillin/nafcillin 150 mg/kg/day div q6h OR cefazolin 100 mg/kg/day IV div q8h (BII) CA-MRSA: clindamycin 30 mg/kg/day IV div q8h or vancomycin 40 mg/kg/day IV q8h (BIII)	Oral antistaphylococcal antibiotic for less severe infection; treatment course for 7–10 days
– Idiopathic (no entry site) in unimmunized infants: pneumococcal or H influenzae type b	Ceftriaxone 50 mg/kg/day q24h OR cefotaxime 100–150 mg/kg/day IV, IM div q8h OR cefuroxime 150 mg/kg/day IV div q8h (AII)	Treatment course for 7–10 days; rule out meningitis; alternative: other 2nd, 3rd, or 4th generation cephalosporins or chloramphenicol
– Periorbital swelling, non-tender (usually associated with sinusitis), sinus pathogens rarely may erode anteriorly causing cellulitis	Ceftriaxone 50 mg/kg/day q24h OR cefotaxime 100–150 mg/kg/day IV, IM div q8h OR cefuroxime 150 mg/kg/day IV div q8h (BIII) ADD clindamycin 30 mg/kg/day IV div q8h for more severe infection with suspect S aureus including CA-MRSA or for chronic sinusitis (covers anaerobes) (AII)	For oral convalescent antibiotic therapy, see Sinusitis, acute; total treatment course of 21 days or 7 days after resolution of symptoms.
Conjunctivitis, acute (Haemophilus and pneumococcus predominantly)	Polymyxin/trimethoprim ophth soln OR polymyxin/bacitracin ophth ointment OR ciprofloxacin ophth soln (CII), for 7–10 days For neonatal infection, see Chapter 5. Steroid-containing therapy only if HSV ruled out	Other topical antibiotics (gentamicin, tobramycin ophth soln erythromycin, besifloxacin, moxifloxacin, norfloxacin, ofloxacin, levofloxacin) may offer advantages for particular pathogens (CII). High rates of resistance to sulfacetamide

Conjunctivitis, herpetic	Trifluridine 1% ophth soln OR acyclovir 3% ophth ointment (BII) Acyclovir PO (60–80 mg/kg/day div qid) has been effective in limited studies (BII).	Refer to ophthalmologist. Recurrences common; corneal scars may form. Topical steroids for keratitis while using topical antiviral solution. Long-term prophylaxis for suppression of recurrent infection with oral acyclovir 20–25 mg/kg/dose (max 400 mg) PO bid (little long-term safety data in children). Assess for neutropenia on long-term therapy; potential risks must balance potential benefits to vision (BIII).
Dacryocystitis	No antibiotic usually needed: oral therapy for more symptomatic infection, based on Gram stain and culture of pus; topical therapy as for conjunctivitis may be helpful	Warm compresses; may require surgical probing of nasolacrimal duct
Endophthalmitis		
NOTE: Subconjunctival/subtenon antibiotics may be required (vancomycin/ceftazidime or clindamycin/gentamicin); steroids commonly used; requires anterior chamber or vitreous tap for microbiological diagnosis.		
– Empiric therapy following open globe injury	Vancomycin 40 mg/kg/day IV div q8h AND ceftazidime 150 mg/kg/day IV div q8h (AIII)	Refer to ophthalmologist; vitrectomy may be necessary for advanced endophthalmitis.
– Staphylococcal	Vancomycin 40 mg/kg/day IV div q8h pending susceptibility testing; oxacillin/nafcillin 150 mg/kg/day IV div q6h if susceptible (AIII)	
– Pneumococcal, meningococcal, *Haemophilus*	Ceftriaxone 100 mg/kg/day IV q24h; penicillin G 250,000 U/kg/day IV div q4h if susceptible (AIII)	Rule out meningitis; treatment course for 10–14 days
– Gonococcal	Ceftriaxone 50 mg/kg q24h IV, IM (AIII)	Treatment course 7 days or longer

C. EYE INFECTIONS (cont)

Clinical Diagnosis	Therapy (evidence grade)	Comments
Endophthalmitis (cont)		
– *Pseudomonas*	Ceftazidime 150 mg/kg/day IV div q8h AND tobramycin 6–7.5 mg/kg/day IM, IV, or amikacin 15–20 mg/kg/day IM, IV div q8h for 10–14 days (AIII)	Cefepime IV, meropenem IV, or imipenem IV are alternatives (no clinical data). Very poor outcomes.
– *Candida*	Intravitreal amphotericin AND fluconazole 10 mg/kg/day IV (AIII)	
Hordeolum (sty) or chalazion	None (topical antibiotic not necessary)	Warm compresses; I&D when necessary
Retinitis		
– CMV For neonatal: See Chapter 5. For HIV-infected children: visit NIH Web site at http://aidsinfo.nih.gov/contentfiles/Pediatric_OI.pdf.	Ganciclovir 10 mg/kg/day IV div q12h for 2 wk (BIII); if needed, continue at 5 mg/kg/day q24h to complete 6 wk total (BIII)	Neutropenia risk increases with duration of therapy. Foscarnet IV and cidofovir IV are alternatives, but demonstrate significant nephrotoxicity. Insufficient data available to recommend valganciclovir extemporaneous suspension. Intravitreal ganciclovir and combination therapy for non-responding, immunocompromised hosts

D. EAR AND SINUS INFECTIONS

Clinical Diagnosis	Therapy (evidence grade)	Comments
Bullous myringitis (see Otitis media, acute)	Believed to be a clinical presentation of acute bacterial otitis media	
Otitis externa		
– Bacterial (swimmer's ear) (P aeruginosa, S aureus, including CA-MRSA)	Topical antibiotics: fluoroquinolone (ciprofloxacin or ofloxacin) with steroid, OR neomycin/polymyxin B/hydrocortisone (BI) Irrigation and cleaning canal of detritus important	Wick moistened with Burow solution, used for marked swelling of canal; to prevent swimmer's ear, 2% acetic acid to canal after water exposure will restore acid pH
– Bacterial (malignant otitis externa) (P aeruginosa)	Ceftazidime 150 mg/kg/day IV div q8h AND tobramycin 6–7.5 mg/kg/day IM (AIII)	Other antipseudomonal antibiotics should also be effective: cefepime IV, meropenem IV or imipenem IV, pip/tazo
– Bacterial furuncle of canal (S aureus, including CA-MRSA)	Standard: oxacillin/nafcillin 150 mg/kg/day IV div q6h OR cefazolin 100 mg/kg/day IV div q8h (BIII) CA-MRSA: clindamycin 30 mg/kg/day IV div q8h or vancomycin 40 mg/kg/day IV q8h (BII)	I&D; antibiotics for cellulitis Oral therapy for mild disease, convalescent therapy: for MSSA: cephalexin; for CA-MRSA: clindamycin, TMP/SMX, OR linezolid (BIII)
– Candida	Fluconazole 5–10 mg/kg/day PO qd for 5–7 days (CIII)	May occur following antibiotic therapy of bacterial external otitis; debride canal
Otitis media, acute		

A note on AOM: The natural history of AOM in different age groups by specific pathogens has not been well defined; therefore, the actual contribution of antibiotic therapy on resolution of disease has also been poorly defined until 2 recent, amoxicillin/clavulanate vs placebo, blinded, prospective studies were published (Hoberman A et al 2011 and Tähtinen P et al 2011) although neither study requested tympanocentesis to define a pathogen. The benefits and risks (including development of antibiotic resistance) of antibiotic therapy for ACM need to be further evaluated before the most accurate advice on the "best" antibiotic can be provided. However, based on available data, for most children, amoxicillin or amoxicillin/clavulanate can be used initially. Considerations for the need for extended antimicrobial activity of amoxicillin/clavulanate include severity of disease, age of child, previous antibiotics, child care attendance, in vitro antibacterial spectrum of antibiotic, and palatability of suspensions. The most current American Academy of Pediatrics guidelines and metaanalyses suggest the greatest benefit with therapy occurs in children with bilateral AOM who are younger than 2 years; for other children, close observation is also an option. Some experts advocate providing a prescription to parents, but waiting 1–2 days before treating mild cases. Although prophylaxis is only rarely indicated, amoxicillin or other antibiotics can be used in one-half the therapeutic dose once or twice daily to prevent infections if the benefits outweigh the risks of development of resistant organisms for that child.

D. EAR AND SINUS INFECTIONS (cont)

Clinical Diagnosis	Therapy (evidence grade)	Comments
Otitis media, acute (cont)		
– Newborns	See Chapter 5.	
– Infants and children (pneumococcus, H influenzae non-type b, Moraxella most common)	Usual therapy: amoxicillin 90 mg/kg/day PO div bid; failures will be caused by either beta-lactamase–producing Haemophilus (or Moraxella) or highly pen-R pneumococcus a) For pen-R pneumococci: high-dosage amoxicillin achieves better middle ear activity than oral cephalosporins. Options include: ceftriaxone IM 50 mg/kg/day q24h for 1–3 doses; OR levofloxacin 20 mg/kg/day PO bid for children ≤5 y, and 10 mg/kg PO qd for children >5 y; OR a macrolide-class antibiotic: azithromycin PO at 1 of 3 dosages: (1) 10 mg/kg on day 1, followed by 5 mg/kg qd on days 2–5, or (2) 10 mg/kg qd for 3 days, or 30 mg/kg once. Caution: up to 40% of pen-R pneumococci are also macrolide-resistant b) For Haemophilus strains that are beta-lactamase–positive, the following oral antibiotics offer better in vitro activity than amoxicillin: amox/clav, cefdinir, cefpodoxime, cefuroxime, ceftriaxone IM, levofloxacin	See Chapter 11 for dosages. High-dosage amoxicillin (90 mg/kg/day) should be used for empiric therapy in most areas, given the prevalence of pen-R pneumococci. The high serum and middle ear fluid concentrations achieved with 45 mg/kg/dose of amoxicillin, combined with a long half-life in middle ear fluid, allow for a therapeutic antibiotic exposure in the middle ear with only twice-daily dosing; high-dose amoxicillin (90 mg/kg/day) with clavulanate (Augmentin-ES) is also available. If data post-PCV13 use document increasing susceptibility to amoxicillin, standard dosage (45 mg/kg/day) can be recommended. Tympanocentesis should be performed in children who fail second-line therapy.
Otitis, chronic suppurative (P aeruginosa, S aureus, including CA-MRSA, and other respiratory tract/skin flora)	Topical antibiotics: fluoroquinolone (ciprofloxacin, ofloxacin, besifloxacin) with or without steroid (BIII) Cleaning of canal, view of tympanic membrane (TM), for patency; cultures important	Presumed middle ear drainage through open TM; possible aminoglycoside toxicity if neomycin-containing topical therapy used Other topical fluoroquinolones with/without steroids available

Mastoiditis, acute (pneumococcus, S aureus, including CA-MRSA; group A streptococcus; Haemophilus rare)	Cefotaxime 150 mg/kg/day div q8h or ceftriaxone 50 mg/kg/day c24h AND clindamycin 40 mg/kg/day IV div q8h (BIII)	Rule out meningitis; surgery as needed for mastoid and middle ear drainage Change to appropriate oral therapy after clinical improvement
Mastoiditis, chronic (see also Chronic suppurative otitis media) anaerobes, Pseudomonas, S aureus (including CA-MRSA)	Antibiotics only for acute superinfections (according to culture of drainage); for Pseudomonas: meropenem 60 mg/kg/day IV div q8h, OR pip/tazo 240 mg/kg/day IV div q4-6h for 1 wk after drainage stops (BIII)	Daily cleansing of ear important; if no response to antibiotics, surgery Alternative: ceftazidime IV (poor anaerobic coverage) Be alert for CA-MRSA.
Sinusitis, acute (H influenzae non-type b, pneumococcus, group A streptococcus, Moraxella)	Same antibiotic therapy as for AOM (amoxicillin 90 mg/kg/day PO div bid) (BIII) Therapy of 14 days may be necessary while mucosal swelling resolves and ventilation is restored.	For more severe symptoms, use high-dosage amoxicillin with clavulanate to increase the likelihood of cure by extending coverage for ampicillin-R H influenzae (BII). Sinus irrigations for severe disease or failure to respond
E. OROPHARYNGEAL INFECTIONS		
Dental abscess	Clindamycin 30 mg/kg/day PO IV, IV div q6-8h OR penicillin G 100-200,000 J/kg/day IV div q6h (AIII)	Amox/clav PO; ampicillin AND metronidazole IV are other options Tooth extraction usually necessary. Erosion of abscess may occur into facial, sinusitis, deep head, and neck compartments
Diphtheria	Erythromycin 40-50 mg/kg/day PO div qid for 14 days OR penicillin G 150,000 L/kg/day IV div q6h; PLUS antitoxin (AIII)	Diphtheria antitoxin (DAT), a horse antisera, is investigational and only available from CDC Emergency Operations Center at 770/488-7100. The investigational protocol and dosages of DAT are provided on the CDC Web site (protocol version 4/30/2009) at http://www.cdc.gov/vaccines/vpd-vac/diphtheria/dat/downloads/protocol_032504.pdf.

E. OROPHARYNGEAL INFECTIONS (cont)

Clinical Diagnosis	Therapy (evidence grade)	Comments
Epiglottitis (aryepiglottitis, supraglottitis; *H influenzae* type b in an unimmunized child); rarely pneumococcus, *S aureus*	Ceftriaxone 50 mg/kg/day IV, IM q24h OR cefotaxime 150 mg/kg/day IV div q8h for 7–10 days	Emergency: provide airway For *S aureus* (causes only 5% of epiglottitis), consider adding clindamycin 40 mg/kg/day IV div q8h.
Gingivostomatitis, herpetic	Acyclovir 80 mg/kg/day PO div qid for 7 days (for severe disease, use IV therapy at 30 mg/kg/day div q8h) (BIII); OR for infants ≥3 mo of age, valacyclovir 50 mg/kg/day PO div bid (crush tablets to create 25 or 50 mg/mL in suspension structured vehicle USP-NF) (CIII)	This is the safe and effective acyclovir dosage for varicella; 75 mg/kg/day div into 5 equal doses has been studied for HSV. Valacyclovir pharmacokinetics have been determined in one pediatric study. Start treatment as soon as oral intake compromised. Consider adding amox/clav or clindamycin for severe disease with oral flora superinfection.
Lemierre syndrome (*Fusobacterium necrophorum*) pharyngitis with internal jugular vein septic thrombosis, postanginal sepsis, necrobacillosis	Empiric: meropenem 60 mg/kg/day div q8h (or 120 mg/kg/day div q8h for CNS metastatic foci) (AIII) OR ceftriaxone 100 mg/kg/day q24h AND metronidazole 40 mg/kg/day div q8h or clindamycin 40 mg/kg/day div q6h (BIII)	Anecdotal reports suggest metronidazole may be effective for apparent failures with other agents. Often requires anticoagulation Metastatic and recurrent abscesses often develop while on active, appropriate therapy, requiring multiple debridements and prolonged antibiotic therapy. Treat until CRP and ESR are normal (AIII).
Peritonsillar cellulitis or abscess (group A streptococcus with mixed oral flora)	Clindamycin 30 mg/kg/day PO, IV, IM div q8H AND cefotaxime 150 mg/kg/day IV div q8h (BIII)	Consider incision and drainage for abscess Alternatives: meropenem or imipenem; pip/tazo; amox/clav for convalescent oral therapy (BIII) No useful data on benefits of steroids

Pharyngitis (group A streptococcus) tonsillopharyngitis	Amoxicillin 50–75 mg/kg/day PO, either qd, bid, or tid for 10 days OR penicillin V 50–75 mg/kg/day PO div bid or tid, OR benzathine penicillin 600,000 units IM for children <27 kg, 1.2 million units IM if >27 kg, as a single dose (AI) For penicillin-allergic children: erythromycin iestolate at 20–40 mg/kg/day PO div bid to qid; or ethylsuccinate at 40 mg/kg/day PO div bid to qid) for 10 days; or azithromycin 12 mg/kg qd for 5 days (AII)	Amoxicillin displays better gastrointestinal absorption than oral phenoxymethyl penicillin; the suspension is better tolerated. These advantages should be balanced by the unnecessary increased spectrum of activity. qd amoxicillin dosage: for children >3 y and <40 kg: 750 mg qd; for those >40 kg, 1,000 mg qd. Meta-analysis suggests that oral cephalosporins are more effective than penicillin for treatment of strep. Clindamycin is also effective. A 5-day treatment course is FDA approved for some oral cephalosporins (cefdinir, cefpodoxime), but longer follow-up for rheumatic fever is important before short-course therapy can be recommended for all streptococcal pharyngitis (CIII).
Retropharyngeal, parapharyngeal, or lateral pharyngeal cellulitis or abscess (mixed aerobic/anaerobic flora)	Clindamycin 40 mg/kg/day IV div q8h AND cefotaxime 150 mg/kg/day IV div q8h or ceftriaxone 50 mg/kg/day IV q24h	Consider I&D; possible airway compromise, mediastinitis Alternatives: meropenem or imipenem (BIII)
Tracheitis, bacterial (S aureus, including CA-MRSA; group A streptococcus; pneumococcus; H influenzae type b, rarely Pseudomonas)	Vancomycin 40 mg/kg/day IV div q8h or clindamycin 40 mg/kg/day IV div q6h AND ceftriaxone 50 mg/kg/day q24h or cefotaxime 150 mg/kg/day div q8h	For susceptible S aureus, oxacillin/nafcillin or cefazolin May represent bacterial superinfection of viral laryngotracheobronchitis

F. LOWER RESPIRATORY TRACT INFECTIONS

Clinical Diagnosis	Therapy (evidence grade)	Comments
Abscess, lung		
– Primary (severe, necrotizing community-acquired pneumonia caused by pneumococcus, *S aureus*, including CA-MRSA, group A streptococcus)	Empiric therapy with ceftriaxone 50–75 mg/kg/day q24h or cefotaxime 150 mg/kg/day div q8h. For severe disease (presumed *S aureus*), ADD clindamycin 40 mg/kg/day div q8h or vancomycin 40 mg/kg/day IV div q8h for 14–21 days or longer (AIII)	For severe CA-MRSA infections, see Chapter 4. Bronchoscopy necessary if abscess fails to drain; surgical excision rarely necessary for pneumococcus, but more important for CA-MRSA and MSSA. For susceptible staph: oxacillin/nafcillin or cefazolin
Primary, putrid (ie, foul-smelling; polymicrobial infection with oral aerobes and anaerobes)	Clindamycin 40 mg/kg/day IV div q8h OR meropenem 60 mg/kg/day IV div q8h for 10 days or longer (AIII)	Alternatives: imipenem IV, or pip/tazo IV, or ticar/clav IV (BIII) Oral step-down therapy with clindamycin or amox/clav (BIII)
Allergic bronchopulmonary aspergillosis	Prednisone 0.5 mg/kg every other day	Larger dosages may lead to tissue invasion by *Aspergillus*.
Aspiration pneumonia (polymicrobial infection with oral aerobes and anaerobes)	Clindamycin 40 mg/kg/day IV div q8h; ADD ceftriaxone 50–75 mg/kg/day q24h or cefotaxime 150 mg/kg/day div q8h for additional *Haemophilus* activity OR meropenem 60 mg/kg/day IV div q8h; for 10 days or longer (BIII)	Alternatives: imipenem IV or pip/tazo IV or ticar/clav IV (BIII) Oral step-down therapy with clindamycin or amox/clav (BIII)
Atypical pneumonia (see *Mycoplasma*, Legionnaire disease)		
Bronchitis (bronchiolitis), acute	For bronchitis/bronchiolitis in children, no antibiotic needed for most cases, as disease is usually viral	
Community-acquired pneumonia (see Pneumonia: Community-acquired on page 54)		

Condition	Therapy	Comments
Cystic fibrosis, acute exacerbation (*P aeruginosa* primarily; also *Burkholderia cepacia*, *Stenotrophomonas maltophilic*, *S aureus*, including CA-MRSA)	Ceftazidime 150–200 mg/kg/day div q6-8h or meropenem 120 mg/kg/day div q6h AND tobramycin 6–10 mg/kg/day IM IV div q6–8h (AIII); Alternatives: imipenem, cefepime, ticar/clav or ciprofloxacin 30 mg/kg/day PO div tid Duration of therapy not well defined: 2–3 wk (EIII) Inhaled antibiotics for both treatment and prevention of infection Tobramycin 300 mg bid, cycling 28 days on therapy, 28 days off therapy, is effective adjunctive therapy between exacerbation. Azithromycin adjunctive therapy recommended only for those with *Pseudomonas* infection	Larger than normal dosages of antibiotics required in most patients with cystic fibrosis; monitor peak serum concentrations of aminoglycosides Cultures with susceptibility testing and synergy testing will help select antibiotics as multidrug resistance is common. Combination therapy may provide synergistic killing and delay the emergence of resistance (CIII). Alternative inhaled antibiotics: aztreonam; colistin
Pertussis	Azithromycin (10 mg/kg/day for 5 days) or clarithromycin (15 mg/kg/day div bid for 7 days) or erythromycin (estolate preferable) 40 mg/kg/day PO div qid; for 14 days (AII) Alternative: TMP/SMX (8 mg/kg/day TMP) div bid for 14 days (BIII)	Azithromycin and clarithromycin are better tolerated than erythromycin (Chapter 5); azithromycin is preferred in young infants to reduce pyloric stenosis risk. The azithromycin dosage that is recommended for infants <1 mo (12 mg/kg/day for 5 days) is FDA approved for streptococcal pharyngitis and is well tolerated and safe for older children. Alternatively, 10 mg/kg on day 1, followed by 5 mg/kg on days 2–5 should also be effective. Provide prophylaxis to family members.

F. LOWER RESPIRATORY TRACT INFECTIONS (cont)

Clinical Diagnosis	Therapy (evidence grade)	Comments
Pneumonia: Community-acquired, bronchopneumonia		
– Mild to moderate illness (overwhelmingly viral, especially in preschool children)	No antibiotic therapy unless epidemiologic, clinical, or laboratory reasons to suspect bacteria or *Mycoplasma*	Broad-spectrum antibiotics may increase risk of subsequent infection with antibiotic-resistant pathogens.
– Moderate to severe illness (pneumococcus; group A streptococcus; *S aureus*, including CA-MRSA; or *Mycoplasma pneumoniae*; or for those with aspiration due to underlying comorbidities, *Haemophilus influenzae*, nontypable)	Empiric therapy: For regions with high PCV13 vaccine use or low pneumococcal resistance to penicillin: ampicillin 200 mg/kg/day div q6h; For regions with low rates of PCV13 use or high pneumococcal resistance to penicillin: ceftriaxone 50–75 mg/kg/day q24h or cefotaxime 150 mg/kg/day div q8h (AI) For suspected CA-MRSA, use vancomycin 40–60 mg/kg/day (AIII) For suspect *Mycoplasma*/atypical pneumonia agents, particularly in school-aged children, ADD azithromycin 10 mg/kg IV, PO once, then decrease dose to 5 mg/kg qd for days 2–5 of treatment (AII)	Tracheal aspirate or bronchoalveolar lavage for Gram stain/culture for severe infection in intubated children Check vancomycin serum concentrations and renal function, particularly at the higher dosage for CA-MRSA. Alternatives to azithromycin for atypical pneumonia include erythromycin IV, PO, or clarithromycin PO, or doxycycline IV, PO for children >7 y, or levofloxacin for post-pubertal older children.

Pneumonia: Community-acquired, lobar consolidation

Pneumococcus (even if immunized), *S aureus*, including CA-MRSA (can cause necrotizing pneumonia) and group A streptococcus Consider *H influenzae* type b in the unimmunized child. *M pneumoniae* may cause lobar pneumonia.	Empiric therapy: For regions with high PCV13 vaccine use or low pneumococcal resistance to penicillin: ampicillin 200 mg/kg/day div q5h For regions with low rates of PCV 3 use or high pneumococcal resistance to penicillin: ceftriaxone 50–75 mg/kg/day q24h or cefotaxime 150 mg/kg/day div q8h (AII); for more severe disease ADD clindamycin 40 mg/kg/day div q8h or vancomycin 40–60 mg/kg/day div q8h for *S aureus* (AIII) For suspect *Mycoplasma*/atypical pneumonia agents, particularly in school-aged children, ADD azithromycin 10 mg/kg IV, PO once, then decrease dose to 5 mg/kg cd for days 2–5 of treatment (AII). Empiric oral outpatient therapy for less severe illness: high dosage amoxicillin 80–100 mg/kg/day PO div q8h (NCTq12h) for *Mycoplasma*, ADD a macrolide as above (EIII).	Change to PO after improvement (decreased fever, no oxygen needed); treat until clinically asymptomatic and chest radiography significantly improved (7–21 days) (BIII) No reported failures of ceftriaxone/cefotaxime for pen-R pneumococcus: no need to add empiric vancomycin for this reason (CIII) Oral therapy for pneumococcus and *Haemophilus* may also be successful with amox/clav, cefdinir, cefpodoxime, or cefuroxime. Levofloxacin is an alternative (BI) but due to cartilage toxicity concerns, should not be first-line therapy.
– Pneumococcal, pen-S	Penicillin G 250,000–400,000 U/kg/day IV div q4–6h for 10 days (BII) or ampicillin 200 mg/kg/day IV divided q6h	After improvement, change to PO amoxicillin 50–75 mg/kg/day PO div tid, or penicillin V 50–75 mg/kg/day div qid
– Pneumococcal, pen-R	Ceftriaxone 75 mg/kg/day q24h or cefotaxime 150 mg/kg/day div q8h for 10–14 d (BII)	Addition of vancomycin has not been required for eradication of pen-R strains. For oral convalescent therapy, high-dosage amoxicillin (100–150 mg/kg/day PO div tid), or clindamycin (30 mg/kg/day PO div tid), or linezolid (30 mg/kg/day PO div tid)

F. LOWER RESPIRATORY TRACT INFECTIONS (cont)

Clinical Diagnosis	Therapy (evidence grade)	Comments
Pneumonia: Community-acquired, lobar consolidation (cont)		
S aureus (including CA-MRSA)	For MSSA: oxacillin/nafcillin 150 mg/kg/day IV div q6h or cefazolin 100 mg/kg/day IV div q8h (AII) For CA-MRSA: vancomycin 60 mg/kg/day; may need addition of rifampin, clindamycin, or gentamicin (AIII) (see Chapter 4)	Check vancomycin serum concentrations and renal function, particularly at the higher dosage (serum trough concentrations of 15 µg/mL) needed for invasive CA-MRSA disease. For life-threatening disease, optimal therapy of CA-MRSA is not defined: add gentamicin and/or rifampin. Linezolid 30 mg/kg/day IV, PO div q8h is another option (follow platelets and WBC weekly).
Pneumonia: with empyema (same pathogens as for community-associated bronchopneumonia) May benefit from chest tube drainage with fibrinolysis or video-assisted thoracoscopic surgery	Empiric therapy: ceftriaxone 50–75 mg/kg/day q24h or cefotaxime 150 mg/kg/day div q8h AND vancomycin 40–60 mg/kg/day IV div q8h (BIII)	Initial therapy based on Gram stain of empyema fluid; typically clinical improvement is slow, with persisting but decreasing "spiking" fever for 2–3 wk. Broad spectrum empiric therapy recommended due to need to provide initial effective therapy for best outcomes.
– Group A streptococcal	Penicillin G 250,000 U/kg/day IV div q4–6h for 10 days (BII)	Change to PO amoxicillin 75 mg/kg/day tid or penicillin V 50–75 mg/kg/day, div qid to tid after clinical improvement (BIII)
– Pneumococcal	(See above, Pneumonia: Community-acquired, lobar consolidation, Pneumococcus)	
– *S aureus* (including CA-MRSA)	For MSSA: oxacillin/nafcillin or cefazolin (AII) For CA-MRSA: use vancomycin 60 mg/kg/day (AIII) (follow serum concentrations and renal function); may need additional antibiotics (see Chapter 4)	For life-threatening disease, optimal therapy of CA-MRSA is not defined: add gentamicin and/or rifampin Oral convalescent therapy for MSSA: cephalexin PO; for CA-MRSA: clindamycin PO Total course for 21 days or longer (AIII) Linezolid 30 mg/kg/day IV, PO div q8h is another option (follow platelets and WBC weekly).

Pneumonia: immunosuppressed, neutropenic host P aeruginosa, other community-associated or nosocomial gram-negative bacilli, S aureus, fungi, AFB, Pneumocystis, viral (adenovirus, CMV, EBV, influenza, RSV, others)	Ceftazidime 150 mg/kg/day IV div q8h and tobramycin 6.0–7.5 mg/kg/day IM, IV div q8h (AII), OR cefepime 150 mg/kg/day div q8h, or meropenem 60 mg/kg/day div q8h (AII) ± tobramycin (BIII); AND if S aureus suspected clinically, ADD vancomycin 40–60 mg/kg/day IV div q8h (AIII)	Biopsy or bronchoalveolar lavage usually needed to determine need for antifungal, antiviral, antimycobacterial treatment. Antifungal therapy usually started if no response to antibiotics in 48–72h (amphotericin, voriconazole, or caspofungin/micafungin—see Chapter 8). Amikacin 15–22.5 mg/kg/day is alternative aminoglycoside. Use 2 active agents for possible bacterial synergy and decreased risk of emergence of resistance (BIII).
– Pneumonia: Interstitial pneumonia syndrome of early infancy	If Chlamydia trachomatis suspected azithromycin 10 mg/kg on day 1, followed by 5 mg/kg/day qd days 2–5 CR erythromycin 40 mg/kg/day PO div qid for 14 days (BII).	Most often respiratory viral pathogens, CMV, or chlamydial; role of Ureaplasma uncertain
– Pneumonia, Nosocomial (health care–associated/ventilator-associated) P aeruginosa, gram-negative enteric bacilli (Enterobacter, Klebsiella, Serratia, Escherichia coli), Acinetobacter, Stenotrophomonas, and gram-positive organisms including CA-MRSA and Enterococcus	Commonly used regimens: Meropenem 60 mg/kg/day div q8h, OR pip/tazo 240–300 mg/kg/day div q6–8h, OR cefepime 150 mg/kg/day div q8h; ± gentamicin 6.0–7.5 mg/kg/day div q8h (AIII); ADD vancomycin 40–60 mg/kg/day div q8h for suspect CA-MFSA (AIII)	For multidrug-resistant gram-negative bacilli, colistin may be required. Empiric therapy should be institution-specific, based on your hospital's nosocomial pathogens and susceptibilities. Pathogens that cause nosocomial pneumonia often have multidrug resistance. Cultures are critical. Empiric therapy also based on child's prior colonization/infection. Aminoglycosides may not achieve therapeutic concentrations in airways.

F. LOWER RESPIRATORY TRACT INFECTIONS (cont)

Pneumonias of other established etiologies
(see Chapter 7 for treatment by pathogen)

Clinical Diagnosis	Therapy (evidence grade)	Comments
– Chlamydia (now Chlamydophila) pneumoniae, C psittaci, or C trachomatis	Azithromycin 10 mg/kg on day 1, followed by 5 mg/kg/day qd days 2–5 or erythromycin 40 mg/kg/day PO div qid; for 14 days	Doxycycline (patients >7 y)
– CMV (immunocompromised host)	Ganciclovir IV 10 mg/kg/day IV div q12h for 2 wk (BIII); if needed, continue at 5 mg/kg/day q24h to complete 4–6 wk total (BIII)	Add IVIG or CMV immune globulin to provide a small incremental benefit (BII). For older children, oral valganciclovir may be used for convalescent therapy (BIII).
– E coli	Ceftriaxone 50–75 mg/kg/day q24h or cefotaxime 150 mg/kg/day div q8h (AII)	For resistant strains (ESBL-producers), use meropenem, imipenem, or ertapenem (AII)
– Enterobacter spp	Cefepime 100 mg/kg/day div q12h or meropenem 60 mg/kg/day div q8h; OR ceftriaxone 50–75 mg/kg/day q24h or cefotaxime 150 mg/kg/day div q8h AND gentamicin 6.0–7.5 mg/kg/day IM, IV div q8h (AIII)	Addition of aminoglycoside to 3rd generation cephalosporins may retard the emergence of constitutive high-level resistance, but concern for inadequate concentration in airways; not needed with cefepime, meropenem, or imipenem
– Francisella tularensis	Gentamicin 6.0–7.5 mg/kg/day IM, IV div q8h for 10 days or longer for more severe disease (AIII); for less severe disease, doxycycline PO (AIII)	Alternatives for oral therapy of mild disease: ciprofloxacin or levofloxacin (BIII) The rate of relapse seems to be higher with tetracycline.
– Fungi (see Chapter 8) – Community-associated pathogens vary by region (eg, coccidioides, histoplasma) – Aspergillus, mucor, others in immunocompromised hosts	For pathogen-specific recommendations, see Chapter 8. For suspected deep fungi in immunocompromised host, treat empirically with a lipid amphotericin B OR voriconazole; biopsy needed to guide therapy	For normal hosts, triazoles (fluconazole, itraconazole, voriconazole) are better tolerated than amphotericin and equally effective for many community-associated pathogens (see Chapter 2). For dosage, see Chapter 8.

– Influenza virus For 2010–2011, seasonal A and B strains were neuraminidase S and adamantane R.	Empiric therapy: 1 y–≤7 y: oseltamivir; for >7 y: oseltamivir OR zanamivir inhaled alone (AIII) For flu B: 1 y–≤7 y: oseltamivir; for >7 y: oseltamivir or zanamivir inhaled (AII)	Adamantanes are amantadine and rimantadine. FluB is intrinsically resistant to adamantanes. For empiric therapy of infants <1 y, limited safety and dosing information exist for oseltamivir. For dosage, see Chapter 9.
– Klebsiella pneumoniae	Ceftriaxone 50–75 mg/kg/day IV, IM q24h OR cefotaxime 150 mg/kg/day IV, IM div q8h (AIII); for ceftriaxone-resistant strains (ESBL strains), use meropenem 60 mg/kg/day IV div q8h (AIII)	For K pneumoniae carbapenemase-producing strains: alternatives include fluoroquinolones or colistin (BIII)
– Legionnaire disease (Legionella pneumophila)	Azithromycin 10 mg/kg IV, PO q24h for 5 days (AIII)	Alternatives: clarithromycin, erythromycin, ciprofloxacin, levofloxacin, doxycycline
– Mycobacteria, nontuberculous (M avium complex most common)	In a normal host: azithromycin PO or clarithromycin PO for 6–12 wk if susceptible For more extensive disease: a macrolide AND rifampin AND ethambutol; ± amikacin or streptomycin (AIII)	Highly variable susceptibilities of different nontuberculous mycobacterial species Check for immunocompromise: HIV or gamma-interferon receptor deficiency
– Mycobacterium tuberculosis (see Tuberculosis)		
– M pneumoniae	Azithromycin 10 mg/kg on day 1, followed by 5 mg/kg/day qd days 2–5, or clarithromycin 15 mg/kg/day div bid for 7–14 days, or erythromycin 40 mg/kg/day PO div qid for 14 days	Mycoplasma often causes self-limited infection and does not require treatment (AIII). For older children, doxycycline Macrolide-resistant strains have recently appeared in the US.
– Paragonimus westermani	See Chapter 10.	
– Pneumocystis jiroveci (previously Pneumocystis carinii)	Mild-moderate disease: TMP/SMX 20 mg of TMP/kg/day PO div qid for 14–21 days (AII); Moderate-severe disease: same dosage of TMP/SMX given IV, each dose over 1h (AI) Use steroid adjunctive treatment for more severe disease (AII).	Alternatives: pentamidine 3–4 mg IV qd, infused over 60–90 min (AII); TMP AND dapsone; OR primaquine AND clindamycin; OR atovaquone Prophylaxis: TMP/SMX 5 mg TMP/kg/day PO daily or 3 times/wk (AII); OR dapsone 1 mg/kg PO qd

F. LOWER RESPIRATORY TRACT INFECTIONS (cont)

Clinical Diagnosis	Therapy (evidence grade)	Comments
Pneumonias of other established etiologies (cont) (see Chapter 7 for treatment by pathogen)		
– P aeruginosa	Ceftazidime 150 mg/kg/day IV div q8h AND tobramycin 6.0–7.5 mg/kg/day IM, IV div q8h (AII). Alternatives: cefepime 150 mg/kg/day div q8h or meropenem 60 mg/kg/day div q8h, OR pip/tazo 240–300 mg/kg/day div q6–8h (AII) ± tobramycin (BIII)	Ciprofloxacin IV, or colistin IV for multidrug-resistant strains
– RSV infection (bronchiolitis, pneumonia)	For immunocompromised hosts: ribavirin aerosol: 6-g vial (20 mg/mL in sterile water), by SPAG-2 generator, over 18–20 h daily for 3–5 days	Treat only for severe disease, immunocompromise, severe underlying cardiopulmonary disease. Ribavirin may also be given systemically (no data on efficacy). Palivizumab is not effective for treatment, only prevention.
Tuberculosis		
– Primary pulmonary disease	Isoniazid (INH) 10–15 mg/kg/day (max 300 mg) PO qd AND rifampin 10–20 mg/kg/day PO qd for 6 mo (max 600 mg) AND PZA 20–40 mg/kg/day PO qd for first 2 mo therapy only (AII) If risk factors present for multidrug resistance, add ethambutol 20 mg/kg/day PO qd OR streptomycin 30 mg/kg/day IV, IM q12h initially.	Contact TB specialist for therapy of drug-resistant TB. Fluoroquinolones may play a role in treating multidrug-resistant strains. Directly observed therapy preferred; after 2 wk of daily therapy, can change to twice weekly dosing double dosage of INH (max 900 mg), PZA (max 2 g), and ethambutol (max 2.5 g); rifampin remains same dosage (10–20 mg/kg/day, max 600 mg) (AII) LP ± CT of head for children ≤2 y to rule out occult, concurrent CNS infection; consider testing for HIV infection (AIII)
– Skin test conversion (latent TB infection)	INH 10–15 mg/kg/day (max 300 mg) PO daily for 9 mo (12 mo for immunocompromised patients) (AIII); treatment with INH at 20–30 mg twice weekly for 9 mo is also effective (AIII)	Single drug therapy if no clinical or radiographic evidence of active disease For exposure to known INH-R but rifampin-S strains, use rifampin 6 mo (AIII)

– Exposed infant <4 y, or immunocompromised patient (high risk of dissemination)	INH 10–15 mg/kg PO daily for 2–3 mo after last exposure with repeat skin test or interferon-gamma release assay test negative (AIII)	If PPD remains negative at 2–3 mo and child well, consider stopping empiric therapy. PPD may not be reliable in immunocompromised patients.

G. CARDIOVASCULAR INFECTIONS

– Bacteremia

– Occult bacteremia (fever without focus), infants <2 mo (group B streptococcus, E coli, Listeria, pneumococcus, meningococcus)	In general, hospitalization with cultures of blood, urine, and CSF; start ampicillin 200 mg/kg/day IV div q6h AND cefotaxime 150 mg/kg/day IV div q8h (AII)	For a nontoxic, febrile infant with good access to medical care; cultures may be obtained of blood, urine, and CSF; ceftriaxone 50 mg/kg IM (lacks Listeria activity) given with outpatient follow-up the next day (Boston Criteria) (BIII); alternative is home without antibiotics if evaluation is negative (Rochester; Philadelphia Criteria) (BI)
– Occult bacteremia (fever without focus) in ages 2–3 mo–36 mo (H influenzae, pneumococcus, meningococcus; increasingly S aureus)	Empiric therapy: If unimmunized, febrile, mild-moderate toxic: after blood culture: ceftriaxone 50 mg/kg IM (BII) If fully immunized (Haemophilus and Pneumococcus) and nontoxic, no routine antibiotic therapy recommended, but: follow closely in case of vaccine failure or meningococcal bacteremia (BII)	Oral convalescent therapy is selected by susceptibility of blood isolate, following response to IM/IV treatment, with CNS and other foci ruled out by exam ± lab tests ± imaging
– H influenzae, type b, non-CNS infections	Ceftriaxone IM/IV OR if beta-lactamase negative, ampicillin IV, followed by oral convalescent therapy (AII)	If beta-lactamase negative: amoxicillin 75–100 mg/kg/day PO div tid (AII) If pos: high-dosage cefixime, ceftibuten, cefdinir PO, or levofloxacin PO (CIII)
– Meningococcus	Ceftriaxone IM/IV or penicillin G IV, followed by oral convalescent therapy (AII)	Amoxicillin 75–100 mg/kg/day PO div tid (AIII)
– Pneumococcus, non-CNS infections	Ceftriaxone IM/IV or penicillin G IV, followed by oral convalescent therapy (AII)	If pen-S: amoxicillin 75–100 mg/kg/day PO div tid (AII) If pen-R: continue ceftriaxone IM, or switch to clindamycin if susceptible (CIII); linezolid or levofloxacin may also be effective (CIII)

G. CARDIOVASCULAR INFECTIONS (cont)

Clinical Diagnosis	Therapy (evidence grade)	Comments
– S aureus	MSSA: nafcillin or oxacillin/nafcillin IV (150–200 mg/kg/day div q6h) ± gentamicin (6 mg/kg/day div q8h) MRSA: vancomycin (40–60 mg/kg/day IV div q8h) ± gentamicin (6 mg/kg/day div q8h) ± rifampin (20 mg/kg/day q12h)	For persisting bacteremia, consider daptomycin 6–8 mg/kg qd (but will not treat pneumonia). For toxic shock syndrome, clindamycin should be added for the initial 48–72h of therapy to decrease toxin production; IVIG may be added to bind circulating toxin (linezolid may also act in this way). Watch for the development of metastatic foci of infection, including endocarditis. If catheter-related, remove catheter.

Endocarditis: Surgical indications: intractable heart failure; persistent uncontrollable infection; large mobile vegetations; peripheral embolism; and valve dehiscence, perforation, rupture or fistula, or a large perivalvular abscess

Clinical Diagnosis	Therapy (evidence grade)	Comments
– Native valve		
– Empiric therapy for presumed endocarditis	Ceftriaxone IV (100 mg/kg q24h) AND gentamicin IV, IM (6 mg/kg/day div q8h) (AII) For severe infection, ADD vancomycin (40–60 mg/kg/day IV div q8h) to cover S aureus (AIII)	Combination (ceftriaxone + gentamicin) provides bactericidal activity against most strains of viridans streptococci, the most common pathogens in infective endocarditis. May administer gentamicin with a qd regimen (CIII). For beta-lactam allergy, use vancomycin 40 mg/kg/day IV div q8h AND gentamicin 6 mg/kg/day IV div q8h.
– Viridans streptococci: Follow echocardiogram for resolution of vegetation (BIII); for beta-lactam allergy: vancomycin		
– Fully susceptible to penicillin	Ceftriaxone 50 mg/kg IV, IM q24h for 4 wk OR penicillin G 200,000 U/kg/day IV div q4–6h for 4 wk (BII); OR penicillin G or ceftriaxone AND gentamicin 6 mg/kg/day IM, IV div q8h for 14 days (AII)	
– Relatively resistant to penicillin	Penicillin G 300,000 U/kg/day IV div q4–6h for 4 wk, or ceftriaxone 100 mg/kg IV q24h for 4 wk; AND gentamicin 6 mg/kg/day IM, IV div q8h for 2 wk (AIII)	Gentamicin is used for the first 2 wk of a total of 4 wk of therapy for relatively resistant strains.

Enterococcus (dosages for both native or prosthetic valve infections)		
– ampicillin-susceptible (gentamicin-S) – ampicillin-resistant (gentamicin-S) – vancomycin-resistant (gentamicin-S)	Ampicillin 300 mg/kg/day IV, IM div q6h or penicillin G 300,000 U/kg/day IV div q4–6h; AND gentamicin 6.0 mg/kg/day IV div q8h; for 4–6 wk (AII) Vancomycin 40 mg/kg/day IV div q8h AND gentamicin 6.0 mg/kg/day IV div q8h; for 4–6 wk (AIII) Daptomycin 6–8 mg/kg/day q24h AND gentamicin 6.0 mg/kg/day IV div q8h; for 4–6 wk (AIII)	Combined treatment with cell-wall active antibiotic plus aminoglycoside used to achieve bactericidal activity For beta-lactam allergy: vancomycin Little data exist in children. Linezolid and quinopristin/dalfopristin are alternatives. For gentamicin-R strains, use streptomycin if susceptible.
– Staphylococci: S aureus, including CA-MRSA; S epidermidis. Consider continuing therapy at end of 6 wk if vegetations persist on echocardiogram	MSSA or MSSE: nafcillin or oxacillin/nafcillin 150–200 mg/kg/day IV div q6h for 6 wk AND gentamicin 6 mg/kg/day div q8h for 14 days CA-MRSA or MRSE: vancomycin 40–60 mg/kg/day IV div q8h AND gentamicin; ADD rifampin 20 mg/kg/day IV div q8–12h	Surgery may be necessary in acute phase; avoid cephalosporins (conflicting data on efficacy). For failures on therapy, consider daptomycin 6–8 mg/kg/day q24h AND gentamicin 6 mg/kg/day div q8h.
– Pneumococcus, gonococcus, group A streptococcus	Penicillin G 200,000 U/kg/day IV div q4–6h for 4 wk; alternatives: ceftriaxone or vancomycin	Ceftriaxone for gonococcus until susceptibilities known For penicillin non-susceptible strains of pneumococcus, use high-dosage penicillin G 300,000 U/kg/day IV div q4–6h or high-dosage ceftriaxone 100 mg/kg IV q24h for 4 wk.
Prosthetic valve/material		
– Viridans streptococci		Follow echocardiogram for resolution of vegetation For beta-lactam allergy: vancomycin
– Fully susceptible to penicillin	Ceftriaxone 100 mg/kg IV, IM q24h for 6 wk OR penicillin G 300,000 U/kg/day IV div q4–6h for 6 wk (AII); OR penicillin G or ceftriaxone AND gentamicin 6.0 mg/kg/day IM, IV div q8h for 14 days (AII)	Gentamicin is used for the first 2 wk of a total of 6 wk of therapy for prosthetic valve/material endocarditis.

G. CARDIOVASCULAR INFECTIONS (cont)

Clinical Diagnosis	Therapy (evidence grade)	Comments
– Prosthetic valve/material (cont)		
– Relatively resistant to penicillin	Penicillin G 300,000 U/kg/day IV div q4–6h for 6 wk, or ceftriaxone 100 mg/kg IV q24h for 6 wk; AND gentamicin 6.0 mg/kg/day IM, IV div q8h for 6 wk (AIII)	Gentamicin is used for all 6 wk of therapy for prosthetic valve/material endocarditis caused by relatively resistant strains.
– Enterococcus (see dosages under Native valve)		
– Staphylococci: *S aureus*, including CA-MRSA; *S epidermidis*. Consider continuing therapy at end of 6 wk if vegetations persist on echocardiogram	MSSA or MSSE: nafcillin or oxacillin/nafcillin 150–200 mg/kg/day IV div q6h AND gentamicin 6 mg/kg/day div q8h AND rifampin 20 mg/kg/day IV div q8–12h IV (AIII) CA-MRSA or MRSE: vancomycin 40–60 mg/kg/day IV div q8h AND gentamicin 6 mg/kg/day div q8h AND rifampin 20 mg/kg/day IV div q8–12h IV (AIII)	Surgery may be necessary in acute phase; avoid cephalosporins (conflicting data on efficacy). For failure to respond in CA-MRSA, consider daptomycin 6–8 mg/kg/day q24h AND gentamicin 6 mg/kg/day div q8h (CIII).

Endocarditis Prophylaxis: Given that (1) endocarditis is rarely caused by dental/GI procedures; and (2) prophylaxis for procedures prevents an exceedingly small number of cases, the risks of antibiotics outweigh the benefits. Highest risk conditions currently recommended for prophylaxis: (1) prosthetic heart valve (or prosthetic material used to repair a valve); (2) previous endocarditis; (3) cyanotic congenital heart disease that is unrepaired (or palliatively repaired with shunts and conduits); (4) congenital heart disease that is repaired but with defects at the site of repair adjacent to prosthetic material; (5) completely repaired congenital heart disease using prosthetic material, for the first 6 mo after repair; or (6) cardiac transplant patients with valvulopathy. Routine prophylaxis no longer is required for children with native valve abnormalities.

– In highest risk patients: dental procedures that involve manipulation of the gingival or periodontal region of teeth	Amoxicillin 50 mg/kg PO 1 h before procedure OR ampicillin or ceftriaxone or cefazolin, all at 50 mg/kg IM/IV 30–60 min before procedure	If penicillin allergy: clindamycin 20 mg/kg PO (60 min before) or IV (30 min before); OR azithromycin 15 mg/kg or clarithromycin 15 mg/kg, 1 h before
– Genitourinary and gastrointestinal procedures	None	No longer recommended

Lemierre syndrome (*Fusobacterium necrophorum*) postanginal sepsis, pharyngitis with internal jugular vein septic thrombosis	Empiric: meropenem 60 mg/kg/day div q8h (or 120 mg/kg/day div q8h for CNS metastatic foci) (AIII) OR ceftriaxone 100 mg/kg/day q24h AND metronidazole 40 mg/kg/day div q8h or clindamycin 40 mg/kg/day div q6h (BIII)	Anecdotal reports suggest metronidazole may be effective for apparent failures with other agents. Metastatic and recurrent abscesses often develop while on active, appropriate therapy, requiring multiple debridements and prolonged antibiotic therapy.

Purulent pericarditis

– Empiric (acute, bacterial: pneumococcus, meningococcus, *S aureus*, group A streptococcus, *H influenzae* type b)	Vancomycin 40 mg/kg/day IV div q8h AND ceftriaxone 50–75 mg/kg/day q24h (AIII) For presumed staphylococcal infection, ADD gentamicin (AIII).	Pericardiocentesis is essential to establish diagnosis. Surgical drainage of pus with pericardial window or pericardiectomy is important to prevent tamponade.
– *S aureus*	For MSSA: oxacillin/nafcillin 150–200 mg/kg/day IV div q6h OR cefazolin 100 mg/kg/day IV div q8h For CA-MRSA: continue vancomycin	Continue therapy with gentamicin; consider use of rifampin in severe cases. Treatment for 3–4 wk.
– *H influenzae* type b in unimmunized children	Ceftriaxone 50 mg/kg/day q24h or cefotaxime 150 mg/kg/day div q8h; for 10–14 days (AIII)	Ampicillin for beta-lactamase–negative strains
– Pneumococcus, meningococcus, group A streptococcus	Penicillin G 200,000 U/kg/day IV, IM div q6h for 10–14 days OR ceftriaxone 50 mg/kg qd for 10–14 days (AIII)	Ceftriaxone or cefotaxime for penicillin-nonsusceptible pneumococci
– Coliform bacilli	Ceftriaxone 50–75 mg/kg/day q24h or cefotaxime 150 mg/kg/day div q8h for 3 wk or longer (AIII)	Alternative drugs depending on susceptibilities; for *Enterobacter, Serratia,* or *Citrobacter* use cefepime or meropenem
– Tuberculous	Isoniazid 10–15 mg/kg/day (max 300 mg) PO qd, IV for 6 mo AND rifampin 10–20 mg/kg/day (max 600 mg) PO qd, IV for 6 mo. ADD PZA 20–40 mg/kg/day PO qd for first 2 mo therapy; if suspected multidrug resistance, also add ethambutol 20 mg/kg/day PO qd (AIII).	Corticosteroids improve survival in adults: prednisone 1 mg/kg/day for 4 wk, then 0.5 mg/kg/day for 4 wk, then 0.25 mg/kg/day for 2 wk, then 0.1 mg/kg/day for 1 wk (AIII)

H. GASTROINTESTINAL INFECTIONS (see Chapter 10 for parasitic infections)

Clinical Diagnosis	Therapy (evidence grade)	Comments
Diarrhea/Gastroenteritis		
Note on E coli and diarrheal disease: Antibiotic susceptibility of E coli varies considerably from region to region. For mild to moderate disease, TMP/SMX may be started as initial therapy, but for more severe disease, and for locations with rates of TMP/SMX resistance greater than 10%–20%, oral 3rd generation cephalosporins (eg, cefixime, cefdinir, or ceftibuten), azithromycin, or ciprofloxacin should be used (AIII). Cultures and antibiotic susceptibility testing are recommended for significant disease (AIII).		
– Empiric therapy of community-associated diarrhea in the USA (E coli [including O157:H7 strains], Salmonella, Campylobacter, and Shigella predominate; Yersinia, and parasites causing <5%; however, viral pathogens are far more common, especially for children <3 y)	Cefixime 8 mg/kg/day PO qd (BII); OR azithromycin 10 mg/kg qd for 3 days (BII)	Alternatives: other oral 3rd generation cephalosporins (eg, cefdinir, ceftibuten); or ciprofloxacin 30 mg/kg/day PO div bid; for 5 days; or rifaximin 600 mg/kg/day tid for 3 days (for nonfebrile, nonbloody diarrhea for children >11 y). Controversy exists regarding treatment of O157:H7 strains, with retrospective data to support either treatment, or withholding treatment.
– Traveler's diarrhea: empiric therapy (E coli, Campylobacter, Salmonella, Shigella, plus many other pathogens including protozoa)	Azithromycin 10 mg/kg qd for 3 days (AII); OR rifaximin 600 mg/day div tid for 3 days (for nonfebrile, nonbloody diarrhea for children ≥12 y) (BII); OR cefixime 8–10 mg/kg qd for 5 days (CII); OR ciprofloxacin 30 mg/kg/day div bid for 5 days (CII)	Susceptibility patterns of E coli, Campylobacter, Salmonella, and Shigella vary widely by country; check country-specific data for departing or returning travelers. Azithromycin preferable to ciprofloxacin for travelers to SE Asia given high prevalence of quinolone-resistant Campylobacter. Rifaximin is less effective than ciprofloxacin for invasive bacterial enteritis; rifaximin may not be as efficacious for Shigella and other enterics in patients with dysentery. Adjunctive therapy with loperamide (antimotility) is not recommended for children <2 y, and should be used only in nonfebrile, non-bloody diarrhea. May shorten symptomatic illness by about 24 h.
– Traveler's diarrhea: prophylaxis		– Prophylaxis: Early self-treatment with agents listed above is preferred over long-term prophylaxis, but may use prophylaxis for a short-term (<14 days) visit to very high-risk region: rifaximin (for older children), azithromycin, or bismuth subsalicylate (BIII)

– Aeromonas hydrophila	Ciprofloxacin 30 mg/kg/day PO div bid for 5 days OR Azithromycin 10 mg/kg qd for 3 days OR cefixime 8 mg/kg/day PO qd (BII)	Not all strains produce enterotoxins and diarrhea; role in diarrhea questioned. Resistance to TMP/SMX about 10%–15%. Choose most narrow spectrum agent based on in vitro susceptibilities.
– Campylobacter jejuni	Azithromycin 10 mg/kg/day for 3 days (BII) or erythromycin 40 mg/kg/day PO div qid for 5 days (BII)	Alternatives: doxycycline or ciprofloxacin (high rate of fluoroquinolone resistance in Thailand and India)
– Cholera	Azithromycin 20 mg/kg once; OR doxycycline 4 mg/kg/day (max 200 mg/day) PO div bid, for all ages	Ciprofloxacin or TMP/SMX (if susceptible)
– Clostridium difficile (antibiotic-associated colitis)	Metronidazole 30 mg/kg/day PO div cid OR vancomycin 40 mg/kg/day PO div qid for 7 days; for relapsing C difficile enteritis, consider pulse therapy (1 wk on/1 wk off for 3–4 cycles) or prolonged tapering therapy	Vancomycin is more effective for severe infection. Many infants and children may have asymptomatic colonization with C difficile. Higher risk of relapse in children with multiple comorbidities.
– E coli		
Enterotoxigenic (etiology of most traveler's diarrhea)	Azithromycin 10 mg/kg qd for 3 days; OR cefixime 8 mg/kg/day PO qd for 5 days	Most illnesses brief and self-limited Alternatives: ciprofloxacin or TMP/SMX Resistance increasing worldwide
Enterohemorrhagic (O157:H7; shiga toxin-producing E coli, etiology of HUS)	Controversy on whether treatment of O157:H7 diarrhea results in more or less toxin-mediated renal damage. For severe infection, therapy as for enterotoxigenic strains above.	Injury to colonic mucosa may lead to invasive bacterial colitis.
Enteropathogenic	Neomycin 100 mg/kg/day PO div q6–8h for 5 days	Most traditional "enteropathogenic" strains are not toxigenic or invasive. Postinfection diarrhea may be problematic.

H. GASTROINTESTINAL INFECTIONS (see Chapter 10 for parasitic infections) (cont)

Clinical Diagnosis	Therapy (evidence grade)	Comments
Diarrhea/Gastroenteritis (cont)		
– Gastritis, peptic ulcer disease (*Helicobacter pylori*)	Triple agent therapy: clarithromycin 7.5 mg/kg/dose 2–3 times each day, AND amoxicillin 40 mg/kg/dose (max 1 g) PO bid AND omeprazole 0.5 mg/kg/dose PO bid 2 wk (BII)	Most data from studies in adults; of effective regimens, no one combination has been shown superior. New, current regimens use 4 drugs (with metronidazole) initially, or with relapse, due to concerns for clarithromycin resistance. Other regimens include bismuth, metronidazole instead of amoxicillin, and other proton pump inhibitors
– Salmonellosis		
Non-typhoid strains	Usually none for self-limited diarrhea For persisting symptomatic infection: azithromycin 10 mg/kg qd for 5–7 days (AII); OR ceftriaxone 75 mg/kg/day IV, IM q24h for 5 days (AII); OR cefixime 20–30 mg/kg/day PO for 14 days (BII); OR for susceptible strains: TMP/SMX (8 mg/kg/day of TMP) PO div bid (AI)	Alternatives: ciprofloxacin 30 mg/kg/day PO div bid for 5–7 days (AI)
Typhoid fever	Azithromycin 10 mg/kg qd for 5–7 days (AII); OR ceftriaxone 75 mg/kg/day IV, IM q24h for 5 days (AII); OR cefixime 20–30 mg/kg/day PO, div q12h for 14 days (BII); OR for susceptible strains: TMP/SMX (8 mg/kg/day of TMP) PO div bid (AI)	Watch for relapse if ceftriaxone used Alternatives: ciprofloxacin 30 mg/kg/day PO div bid for 5–7 days (AI)
– Shigellosis	Cefixime 8 mg/kg/day PO qd for 5 days (AII); OR azithromycin 12 mg/kg PO on day 1, followed by 6 mg/kg daily for 4 days (AII); OR ciprofloxacin 30 mg/kg/day PO div bid (BII)	Alternatives for susceptible strains: TMP/SMX (8 mg/kg/day of TMP) PO bid for 5 days; OR ampicillin (not amoxicillin) Ceftriaxone effective IM, IV if parenteral therapy necessary. Avoid antiperistaltic drugs. Treat to decrease communicability, even if symptoms resolving.

– Yersinia enterocolitica	Antimicrobial therapy probably not of value for mild disease in normal hosts TMP/SMX PO, IV; OR ciprofloxacin PO, IV (BIII)	Alternatives: ceftriaxone or gentamicin May mimic appendicitis. Limited clinical data exist on oral therapy.
Intra-abdominal Infection (abscess, peritonitis secondary to bowel/appendix contents)		
– Appendicitis; bowel-associated (enteric gram-negative bacilli, Bacteroides spp, Enterococcus spp, increasingly Pseudomonas)	Meropenem 60 mg/kg/day IV div q8h or imipenem 60 mg/kg/day IV div q6h; OR pip/tazo 240 mg piperacillin/kg/day div q6h; for 7–10 days or longer if suspicion of persisting intra-abdominal abscess (AI) Data support IV outpatient therapy or oral step-down therapy when clinically improved	Many other regimens may be effective, including ampicillin 150 mg/kg/day div q8h AND gentamicin 6–7.5 mg/kg/day IV, IM div q8h AND clindamycin 30 mg/kg/day IV, IM div q8h or metronidazole 40 mg/kg/day IV div q8h; OR ceftriaxone 50 mg/kg q24h AND metronidazole 40 mg/kg/day IV div q8h. Gentamicin demonstrates poor activity at low pH; surgical source control is critical to achieve cure.
– Tuberculosis, abdominal (Mycobacterium bovis, from unpasteurized dairy products)	INH 10–15 mg/kg/day (max 300 mg) PO qd for 5 mo AND rifampin 10–20 mg/kg/day (max 600 mg) PO qd for 6 mo M bovis is resistant to PZA. If risk factors are present for multidrug resistance (eg, poor adherence to previous therapy), add ethambutol 20 mg/kg/day PO qd OR a fluoroquinolone (moxifloxacin or levofloxacin)	Directly observed therapy preferred; after 2+ wk of daily therapy, can change to twice weekly dosing double dosage of INH (max 900 mg); rifampin remains same dosage (10–20 mg/kg/day, max 600 mg) (AII) LP = CT of head for children ≤2 y with active disease to rule out occult, concurrent CNS infection (AIII)
Perirectal abscess (Bacteroides spp other anaerobes, enteric bacilli, and S aureus predominate)	Clindamycin 30–40 mg/kg/day IV div q8h AND cefotaxime or ceftriaxone or gentamicin (BIII)	Surgical drainage alone may be curative.

H. GASTROINTESTINAL INFECTIONS (see Chapter 10 for parasitic infections) (cont)

Clinical Diagnosis	Therapy (evidence grade)	Comments
Diarrhea/Gastroenteritis (cont)		
Peritonitis – Peritoneal dialysis indwelling catheter infection (staphylococcal; enteric gram-negatives; yeast)	Antibiotic added to dialysate in concentrations approximating those attained in serum for systemic disease (eg, 4 μg/mL for gentamicin; 25 μg/mL for vancomycin, 125 μg/mL for cefazolin, 25 μg/mL for ciprofloxacin, etc) after a larger loading dose (AII)	Selection of antibiotic based on organism isolated from peritoneal fluid; systemic antibiotics if there is accompanying bacteremia/fungemia
– Primary (pneumococcus)	Ceftriaxone 50 mg/kg/day q24h, or cefotaxime 150 mg/kg/day div q8h; if penicillin-S, then penicillin G 150,000 U/kg/day IV div q6h; for 7–10 days (AII)	Other antibiotics according to culture and susceptibility tests

I. GENITAL AND SEXUALLY TRANSMITTED INFECTIONS

Consider testing for HIV and other STIs in a child with one documented STI; consider sexual abuse in prepubertal children. The most recent CDC STI treatment guidelines are posted online at http://www.cdc.gov/std/treatment/.

Clinical Diagnosis	Therapy (evidence grade)	Comments
Chancroid (*Haemophilus ducreyi*)	Azithromycin 1 g PO as single dose OR ceftriaxone 250 mg IM as single dose	Alternative: erythromycin 1.5 g/day PO div tid for 7 days OR ciprofloxacin 1,000 mg PO qd, div bid for 3 days
C trachomatis (cervicitis, urethritis)	Azithromycin 20 mg/kg (max 1 g) PO for 1 dose; OR doxycycline (patients >7 y) 40 mg/kg/day (max 200 mg/day) PO div bid for 7 days	Alternatives: erythromycin 2 g/day PO div qid for 7 days; OR levofloxacin 500 mg PO q24h for 7 days
Epididymitis (associated with positive urine cultures and STIs)	Ceftriaxone 50 mg/kg/day q24h for 7–10 days AND (for older children) doxycycline 200 mg/day div bid	Microbiology not well studied in children; in infants, also associated with urogenital tract anomalies. Treat infants for *S aureus* and *E coli*; may resolve spontaneously; in STI, caused by *Chlamydia* and gonococcus.

Gonorrhea		
– Newborns	See Chapter 5.	
– Genital infections (uncomplicated vulvovaginitis, cervicitis, urethritis, or proctitis)	Ceftriaxone 250 mg IM for 1 dose (regardless of weight); OR cefixime 400 mg PO for 1 dose; AND test/treat for chlamydia	Cephalosporins used due to the prevalence of pen-R strains. Azithromycin 2 g PO for 1 dose is an option, but fluoroquinolones are no longer recommended due to resistance.
– Pharyngitis	Ceftriaxone 250 mg IM for 1 dose	
– Disseminated gonococcal infection	Ceftriaxone 50 mg/kg/day IM, IV q24h (max: 1 g); convalescent oral therapy with cefixime PO; total course for 7 days	No studies in children: increase dosage for meningitis.
Granuloma inguinale (Donovanosis, Klebsiella granulomatis, formerly Calymmatobacterium)	Doxycycline 4 mg/kg/day div bid, (max 200 mg/day) PO for ≥1 days until esions completely healed	Primarily in tropical regions of India, Pacific, and Africa Option: azithromycin 1 g PO once weekly for 3 wk
Herpes simplex virus, genital infection	Acyclovir 20–25 mg/kg/dose (max 400 mg) PO tid for 7–10 days (first episode, AII); for more severe infection: acyclovir 15 mg/kg/day IV div q8h as 1 h infusion (AII) For recurrent episodes: treat as above with acyclovir PO, immediately when symptoms begin, for 5 days For suppression: acyclovir 20–25 mg/kg/dose (max 400 mg) PO bid; OR valacyclovir 25 mg/kg/dose PO qd (little long-term safety data in children; no efficacy data)	Alternatives: valacyclovir 25 mg/kg/dose of extemporaneous suspension (directions on package label), max 1.0 g, PO bid for 7–10 days; famciclovir (adult dose) 250 mg PO tid for 7–10 days For suppression: valacyclovir 1.0 g qd for adults
Lymphogranuloma venereum (C trachomatis)	Doxycycline 4 mg/kg/day (max 200 mg/day) PO (patients >7 y) div bid for 21 days, OR erythromycin 2 g/day PO div qid; for ≥21 days	Azithromycin 1.0 g PO once weekly for 3 wk

I. GENITAL AND SEXUALLY TRANSMITTED INFECTIONS (cont)

Clinical Diagnosis	Therapy (evidence grade)	Comments
Pelvic inflammatory disease (*Chlamydia*, gonococcus, plus anaerobes)	Cefoxitin 2 g IV q6h; AND doxycycline 200 mg/day PO or IV div bid; OR clindamycin 900 mg IV q8h and gentamicin 1.5 mg/kg IV, IM q8h for 14 days	Drugs given IV until clinical improvement for 24 h, followed by doxycycline 200 mg/day PO div bid AND clindamaycin 1800 mg/day PO div qid to complete 14 days of therapy Optional regimen: ceftriaxone 250 mg IM for 1 dose AND doxycycline 200 mg/day PO div bid; WITH/WITHOUT metronidazole 1 g/day PO div bid; for 14 days
Syphilis (test for HIV)		
– Congenital	See Chapter 5.	
– Neurosyphilis (positive CSF VDRL or CSF pleocytosis with serologic diagnosis of syphilis)	Crystalline penicillin G 200–300,000 U/kg/day div q6h for 10–14 days (AIII)	
– Primary, secondary	Benzathine penicillin G 50,000 U/kg (max 2,400,000 U) IM as a single dose (AIII); do not use benzathine-procaine penicillin mixtures	Follow-up serologic tests at 6, 12, and 24 mo; 15% may remain seropositive despite adequate treatment. If allergy to penicillin: doxycycline (patients >7 y) 4 mg/kg/day (max 200 mg) PO bid for 14 days CSF exam should be obtained for children being treated for primary or secondary syphilis to rule out asymptomatic neurosyphilis. Test for HIV.
– Syphilis of <1 y duration, without clinical symptoms (early latent syphilis)	Benzathine penicillin G 50,000 U/kg (max 2,400,000 U) IM as a single dose (AIII)	Alternative if allergy to penicillin: doxycycline (patients >7 y) 4 mg/kg/day (max 200 mg/day) PO div bid for 14 days
– Syphilis of >1 y duration, without clinical symptoms (late latent syphilis) or syphilis of unknown duration	Benzathine penicillin G 50,000 U/kg (max 2,400,000 U) IM weekly for 3 doses (AIII)	Alternative if allergy to penicillin: doxycycline (patients >7 y) 4 mg/kg/day (max 200 mg/day) PO div bid for 28 days Look for neurologic, eye, and aortic complications of tertiary syphilis.

Trichomoniasis	Metronidazole 2 g PO as a single dose, OR 500 mg PO bid for 7 days	Tinidazole 50 mg/kg (max 2 g) PO for 1 dose twice daily for 7 days
Urethritis, nongonococcal (see page 71 for gonorrhea therapy)	Azithromycin 20 mg/kg (max 1 g) PO for 1 dose, OR doxycycline (patients >7 y) 40 mg/kg/day (max 200 mg/day) PO div bid for 7 days (All)	Erythromycin, levofloxacin, or ofloxacin
Vaginitis		
– Bacterial vaginosis	Metronidazole 500 mg PO twice daily for 7 days or metronidazole vaginal gel (0.75%) qd for 5 days	Alternative: tinidazole 1 g PO qd for 5 days, OR clindamycin 300 mg PO bid for 7 days or clindamycin vaginal cream for 7 days Relapse common Caused by synergy of *Gardnerella* with anaerobes
– Candidiasis, vulvovaginal	Fluconazole 5 mg/kg PO (max 150 mg) for 1 dose; topical treatment with azole creams (see Comments)	Many topical vaginal azole agents are available without prescription (eg, butoconazole, clotrimazole, miconazole, tioconazole) and some require a prescription for unique agents or unique dosing regimens (terconazole, butoconazole).
– *Shigella*	Cefixime 8 mg/kg/day PO qd; OR ciprofloxacin 30 mg/kg/day PO div bid for 5 days	50% have bloody discharge; usually not associated with diarrhea.
– *Streptococcus*, group A	Penicillin V 50–75 mg/kg/day PO div tid for 10 days	Amoxicillin 50–75 mg/kg/day PO div tid

J. CENTRAL NERVOUS SYSTEM INFECTIONS

Clinical Diagnosis	Therapy (evidence grade)	Comments
Abscess, brain (respiratory tract flora, skin flora, or bowel flora, depending on the pathogenesis of infection based on underlying comorbid disease and origin of bacteremia)	Until etiology established, cover normal flora of respiratory tract, skin, and/or bowel, based on individual patient evaluation: meropenem 120 mg/kg/day div q8h (AIII); OR nafcillin 150–200 mg/kg/day IV div q6h AND cefotaxime 200–300 mg/kg/day IV div q6h or ceftriaxone 100 mg/kg/day IV q24h AND metronidazole 30 mg/kg/day IV div q8h (BIII); for 2–3 wk after successful drainage (depending on pathogen, size of abscess, and response to therapy); longer course if no surgery (3–6 wk) (BIII)	Surgery for abscesses ≥2 cm diameter If CA-MRSA suspected, ADD vancomycin 60 mg/kg/day IV div q8h ± rifampin 20 mg/kg/day IV div q12h, pending culture results If secondary to chronic otitis, include meropenem or cefepime in regimen for anti-*Pseudomonas* activity. Follow abscess size by CT. For treatment of rare and unusual pathogens that present with symptoms of encephalitis, see IDSA guidelines on encephalitis (2008).
Encephalitis		
– Amebic (*Naegleria fowleri, Balamuthia mandrillaris,* and *Acanthamoeba*)	See Chapter 10 (parasitic pathogens), Amebiasis.	
– CMV	Not well studied in children. Consider ganciclovir (10–20 mg/kg/day IV div q12h); for severe immunocompromise, ADD foscarnet.	Toxicity not well defined over 10 mg/kg/day
– Enterovirus	Supportive therapy; no antivirals currently available	
– EBV	Not well studied. Consider ganciclovir (10–20 mg/kg/day IV div q12h) or acyclovir (60 mg/kg/day IV div q8h)	Efficacy and toxicity of high-dose ganciclovir and acyclovir are not well defined; some experts recommend against antiviral treatment.
– Herpes simplex virus	Acyclovir 60 mg/kg/day IV div q8h (1 h infusion time) for 21 days	(See Chapter 5 for neonatal infection.) Toxicity not well defined at this high dosage; follow closely for hematologic toxicity; FDA has approved acyclovir at this dosage for encephalitis for children up to 12 y
– Toxoplasma	See Chapter 10.	

– Arbovirus (flaviviruses—West Nile, St Louis encephalitis; tickborne encephalitis; togavirus—Western equine encephalitis, Eastern equine encephalitis; bunyavirus—LaCrosse encephalitis, California encephalitis)	Supportive therapy	Investigational only (antiviral, interferon, immune globulins)

Meningitis, bacterial, community-associated

NOTES

- In areas where pen-R pneumococci exist (>5% of invasive strains), initial empiric therapy for suspect pneumococcal meningitis should be with vancomycin AND cefotaxime or ceftriaxone until susceptibility test results are available.
- Dexamethasone (0.6 mg/kg/day IV div q6h for 2 days) as an adjunct to antibiotic therapy decreases hearing deficits and other neurologic sequelae in adults and children (for *Haemophilus* and pneumococcus; not studied for meningococcus or *E coli*). The first dose of dexamethasone is given before or concurrent with the first dose of antibiotic; probably little benefit if given ≥1 h after the antibiotic.
- Preliminary data (we hope to see these confirmed before we recommend) suggest that oral glycerol (85% solution, 1 mL to contain 1 g of glycerol) given at 1.5 g (1.5 mL) per kg (max 25 mL) every 6 h for 48 h, may decrease neurologic sequelae.

– Empiric therapy	Cefotaxime 200–300 mg/kg/day IV div q6h, or ceftriaxone 100 mg/kg/day IV q24h; AND vancomycin 60 mg/kg/day IV div q8h (AII)	If Gram stain or cultures demonstrate a pathogen other than pneumococcus, vancomycin is not needed; vancomycin used empirically only for possible pen-R pneumococcus.
– *H influenzae* type b	Cefotaxime 200–300 mg/kg/day IV div q6h, or ceftriaxone 100 mg/kg/day IV q24h; for 10 days (AI)	Alternative: ampicillin 200–400 mg/kg/day IV div q6h (for beta-lactamase negative strains) OR chloramphenicol 100 mg/kg/day IV div q6h
– Meningococcus (*Neisseria meningitidis*)	Penicillin G 250,000 U/kg/day IV div q4h; or ceftriaxone 100 mg/kg/day IV q24h, or cefotaxime 200 mg/kg/day IV div q6h; treatment course for 7 days (AI)	Meningococcal prophylaxis: rifampin 10 mg/kg PO q12h for 4 doses OR ceftriaxone 125–250 mg IM once OR ciprofloxacin 500 mg PO once (adolescents and adults)
– Neonatal	See Chapter 5.	

J. CENTRAL NERVOUS SYSTEM INFECTIONS (cont)

Clinical Diagnosis	Therapy (evidence grade)	Comments
Meningitis, bacterial, community-associated (cont)		
– Pneumococcus (*S pneumoniae*)	For penicillin- and cephalosporin-susceptible strains: penicillin G 250,000 U/kg/day IV div q4–6h, OR ceftriaxone 100 mg/kg/day IV div q24h or cefotaxime 200–300 mg/kg/day IV div q6h; for 10 days (AI) For pen-R pneumococci: continue the combination of vancomycin and cephalosporin IV for total course (AIII)	Some pneumococci may be resistant to penicillin but susceptible to cefotaxime and ceftriaxone and may be treated with the cephalosporin alone. Test-of-cure LP helpful in those with pen-R pneumococci
Meningitis, TB (*M tuberculosis; M bovis*)	For non-immunocompromised children: INH 15 mg/kg/day PO, IV div q12–24h AND rifampin 15 mg/kg/day PO, IV, div q12–24h for 12 mo AND PZA 30 mg/kg/day PO div q12–24h for first 2 mo of therapy, AND streptomycin 30 mg/kg/day IV, IM div q12h for first 4–8 wk of therapy until susceptibility test results available. For recommendations for drug-resistant strains, and treatment of TB in HIV-infected patients, visit the CDC Web site for TB: http://www.cdc.gov/tb/.	Hyponatremia from inappropriate ADH secretion is common; ventricular drainage may be necessary for obstructive hydrocephalus. Corticosteroids (can use the same dexamethasone dose as for bacterial meningitis, 0.6 mg/kg/day IV div q6h) for 2–4 wk until neurologically stable, then taper dose for 1–3 mo to decrease neurologic complications and improve prognosis by decreasing the incidence of infarction.
Shunt infections: The use of antibiotic-impregnated shunts has decreased the frequency of this infection. Shunt removal usually necessary for cure.		
– Empiric therapy pending Gram stain and culture	Vancomycin 60 mg/kg/day IV div q8h, AND ceftriaxone 100 mg/kg/day IV div q24h (AII)	If Gram stain shows only gram-positive cocci, can use vancomycin alone. Ceftazidime should be used instead of ceftriaxone if *Pseudomonas* is suspected.
– *S epidermidis* or *S aureus*	Vancomycin (for *S epidermidis* and for CA-MRSA) 60 mg/kg/day IV div q8h; OR nafcillin (if organisms susceptible) 150–200 mg/kg/day AND (if severe infection, or slow response) gentamicin or rifampin; for 10–14 days (AIII)	Shunt removal usually necessary; may need to treat with ventriculostomy until ventricular CSF cultures negative; obtain CSF cultures at time of shunt replacement, continue therapy an additional 48–72 h pending cultures.

– Gram-negative bacilli	Empiric therapy with meropenem 120 mg/kg/day IV div q8h OR cefepime 150 mg/kg/day IV div q8h (AIII) For E coli: ceftriaxone 100 mg/kg/day IV div IV q12h OR cefotaxime 200–300 mg/kg/day IV div q6h; ADD gentamicin 6–7.5 mg/kg/day IV until CSF sterile; for 21 days or longer	Remove shunt. Select appropriate therapy based on in vitro susceptibilities. Intrathecal therapy with aminoglycosides not routinely necessary with highly active beta-lactam therapy and shunt removal.

K. URINARY TRACT INFECTIONS

NOTE: Antibiotic susceptibility profiles of E coli, the most common cause of urinary tract infection, vary considerably. For mild disease, TMP/SMX may be started as initial therapy if local susceptibility ≥80% and a 20% failure rate is acceptable. For moderate to severe disease (possible pyelonephritis), obtain cultures and begin oral 2nd or 3rd generation cephalosporins (cefuroxime, cefaclor, cefprozil, cefixime, ceftibuten, cefdinir, cefpodoxime), ciprofloxacin PO, or ceftriaxone IM. Antibiotic susceptibility testing will help direct your therapy to the most narrow spectrum agent.

Cystitis, acute (E coli)	For mild disease: TMP/SMX (8 mg/kg/day of TMP) PO bid for 3 days For moderate to severe disease: cefixime 8 mg/kg/day PO qd; OR ceftriaxone 50 mg/kg IM q24h for 3–5 days (with normal anatomy) (BII); follow-up culture after 36–48 h treatment ONLY if still symptomatic	Alternative: amoxicillin 30 mg/kg/day PO div tid if susceptible (BII); ciprofloxacin 15–20 mg/kg/day PO div bid for otherwise resistant organisms
Nephronia, lobar E coli and other enteric rods (also called focal bacterial nephritis)	Ceftriaxone 50 mg/kg/day IM/I / q24h Duration depends on resolution of cellulitis vs development of abscess (10–21 days) (AIII).	Invasive, consolidative parenchymal infection; complication of pyelonephritis, can evolve into renal abscess.
Pyelonephritis, acute (E coli)	Ceftriaxone 50 mg/kg/day IV, IM q24h OR gentamicin 5–6 mg/kg/day IV, IM q24h; switch to oral therapy following clinical response (BII). If organisms resistant to amoxicillin and TMP/SMX, use an oral 2nd or 3rd generation cephalosporin (BII); if cephalosporin-R, can use ciprofloxacin PO 30 mg/kg/day div q12h (BIII); for 7–10 days total (depending on response to therapy).	If bacteremia documented, and infant is <2–3 mo, rule out meningitis and treat 14 days IV or IM (AIII). Aminoglycosides at any dose are more nephrotoxic than beta-lactams (AI).

K. URINARY TRACT INFECTIONS (cont)

Clinical Diagnosis	Therapy (evidence grade)	Comments
Recurrent urinary tract infection, prophylaxis	Only for those with grade III–V reflux, or with recurrent febrile UTI: TMP/SMX (2 mg/kg/dose of TMP) PO qd OR nitrofurantoin 1–2 mg/kg PO qd at bedtime; more rapid resistance may develop using beta-lactams (BII)	Prophylaxis no longer recommended for patients with grade I–II reflux and no evidence of renal damage. Early treatment of new infections is recommended for these children. Resistance eventually develops to every antibiotic; follow resistance patterns for each patient.

L. MISCELLANEOUS SYSTEMIC INFECTIONS

Clinical Diagnosis	Therapy (evidence grade)	Comments
Actinomycosis	Penicillin G 250,000 U/kg/day IV div q6h, or ampicillin 150 mg/kg/day IV div q8h until improved (often up to 6 wk); then long-term convalescent therapy with penicillin V 100 mg/kg/day (up to 4 g/day) PO for 6–12 mo (AII)	Surgery as indicated Alternatives: amoxicillin, clindamycin, erythromycin; ceftriaxone IM/IV, doxycycline for children >7 y
Anaplasmosis (human granulocytotropic anaplasmosis), *Anaplasma phagocytophilum*	Doxycycline 4 mg/kg/day IV, PO (max 200 mg/day) div bid for 7–10 days (regardless of age) (AIII)	For mild disease, consider rifampin 20 mg/kg/day PO bid for 7–10 days (BIII).
Anthrax, sepsis/pneumonia (inhalation), cutaneous, gastrointestinal	For bioterror-associated infection (regardless of age): ciprofloxacin 20–30 mg/kg/day IV div q12h, OR levofloxacin 16 mg/kg/day IV div q12h not to exceed 250 mg/dose (AIII)	On convalescence, can use oral ciprofloxacin or doxycycline; if susceptible, can use penicillin, amoxicillin, or clindamycin. For community-associated infection, amoxicillin (75 mg/kg/day div q8h) or doxycycline for children >7 y should be effective.

Appendicitis (see Peritonitis)		
Brucellosis	Doxycycline 4 mg/kg/day PO (max 200 mg/day) div b.d (for children >7 y) AND rifampin (15–20 mg/kg/day div q12h) BIII); OR (for children <8 y) TMP/SMX (10 mg/kg/day of TMP) IV, PO div q12h AND rifampin (15–20 mg/kg/day d.v q12h) BIII); for 4–8 wk	Combination therapy with rifampin will decrease the risk of relapse. ADD gentamicin 6–7.5 mg/kg/day IV, IM div q8h for the first 1–2 wk of therapy to further decrease risk of relapse (BIII), particularly for endocarditis, osteomyelitis, or meningitis. Prolonged treatment for 4–6 mo and surgical debridement may be necessary for deep infections (AIII).
Cat-scratch disease *(Bartonella henselae)*	Supportive (incision and drainage of infected lymph node); azithromycin 12 mg/kg/day PO qd for 5 days shortens the duration of adenopathy (AIII)	This dosage of azithromycin has been documented to be safe and effective for streptococcal pharyngitis, and may offer greater deep tissue exposure than the dosage studied by Bass et al, and used for otitis media. No prospective data exist for invasive infections: gentamicin (for 14 days) AND TMP/SMX AND rifampin for hepatosplenic disease and osteomyelitis (AIII). For CNS infection, use cefotaxime AND gentamicin ± TMP/SMX (AIII). Alternatives: ciprofloxacin, doxycycline
Chickenpox/Shingles (varicella-zoster virus)	Acyclovir 30 mg/kg/day IV div q8h if severe, or 80 mg/kg/day PO div qic, depending on severity; for 5 days (AI)	See Chapter 9; therapy for 10 days in immunocompromised children. Famciclovir can be made into a suspension with 25 mg and 100 mg sprinkle capsules. See Chapter 9 for dosages by body weight. No treatment data in children (CIII).
Ehrlichiosis (human monocytotropic ehrlichiosis, caused by *Ehrlichia chaffeensis*, and human ehrlichiosis Ewingii, caused by *Ehrlichia ewingii*)	Doxycycline 4 mg/kg/day IV, PO civ bid (max 100 mg/dose) for 7–10 days (regardless of age) (AIII)	For mild disease, consider rifampin 20 mg/kg/day PO bid (max 300 mg/dose) for 7–10 days (BIII)

L. MISCELLANEOUS SYSTEMIC INFECTIONS (cont)

Clinical Diagnosis	Therapy (evidence grade)	Comments
Febrile neutropenic patient (empiric therapy of invasive infection: *Pseudomonas*, enteric gram-negative bacilli, staphylococci, streptococci, yeast, fungi)	Cefepime 150 mg/kg/day div q8h (AI); or meropenem 60 mg/kg/day div q8h (AII); OR ceftazidime 150 mg/kg/day IV div q8h AND tobramycin 6 mg/kg/day IV q8h (AII) ADD vancomycin 40 mg/kg/day IV div q8h if methicillin-resistant *S aureus* or coag-negative staph suspected (eg, central catheter infection) (AII) ADD metronidazole to ceftazidime or cefepime if colitis or other deep anaerobic infection suspected (AIII)	Alternatives: other anti-*Pseudomonas* beta-lactams (imipenem, pip/tazo) AND anti-staphylococcal antibiotics If no response in 4-7 days and no bacterial etiology demonstrated, consider additional empiric therapy with antifungals (BII); dosages and formulations outlined in Chapter 8 For low-risk patients with close follow-up, oral therapy with amox/clav and ciprofloxacin may be used.
Human immunodeficiency virus infection	See Chapter 9.	
Infant botulism	Botulism immune globulin for infants (BabyBIG) 50 mg/kg IV for 1 dose; BabyBIG can be obtained from the California State Health Department: 510/231-7600 or at http://www.infantbotulism. org ($45,300 for a single dose, August 2011) (AI)	http://www.infantbotulism.org/ provides information for physicians and parents. Web site organized by the California Dept of Public Health (accessed 8/28/2011). Aminoglycosides should be avoided as they potentiate the neuromuscular effect of botulinum toxin.
Kawasaki syndrome	No antibiotics; IVIG 2 g/kg as single dose (AI); may need to repeat dose in up to 15% of children for persisting fever that lasts 24 hours after completion of the IVIG infusion (AII). For subsequent relapse, consult an infectious disease physician.	Aspirin 80–100 mg/kg/day qid in acute, febrile phase; once afebrile for 24–48 h, initiate low dosage (3–5 mg/kg/day) aspirin therapy for 6–8 wk (assuming echocardiogram is normal) Role of corticosteroids and infliximab for IVIG-resistant Kawasaki disease under investigation
Leprosy (Hansen disease)	Dapsone 1 mg/kg/day PO qd AND rifampin 10 mg/kg/day PO qd; ADD (for multibacillary disease) clofazimine 1 mg/kg/day PO qd; for 12 mo for paucibacillary disease; for 24 mo for multibacillary disease (AII)	Consult the HRSA (National Hansen's Disease Program) at http://www.hrsa.gov/hansensdisease/ for advice about treatment and free antibiotics: 800/642-2477.

Leptospirosis	Penicillin G 250,000 U/kg/day IV, IM div q6h, or ceftriaxone 50 mg/kg/day q24h; for 7 days (BII) For mild disease, doxycycline (>7 y of age) 4 mg/kg/day (max 200 mg/day) PO div bid for 7–10 days (BII)	Alternative: azithromycin 20 mg/kg on day one, 10 mg/kg on days 2 and 3; OR amoxicillin for children ≤7 y of age with mild disease
Lyme disease (Borrelia burgdorferi)	Neurologic evaluation, including LP, if there is clinical suspicion of CNS involvement	
– Early localized disease	>7 y of age: doxycycline 4 mg/kg/day (max 200 mg/day) PO div bid for 14–21 days (AII) ≤7 y of age: amoxicillin 50 mg/kg/day (max 1.5 g/day) PO div tid for 14–21 days (AII)	Alternative: erythromycin 30 mg/kg/day PO div tid
– Early disseminated disease		
Arthritis (no CNS disease)	Oral therapy as outlined above; for 28 days (AIII)	Persistent or recurrent joint swelling after treatment: repeat a 4-wk course of oral antibiotics or give ceftriaxone 75–100 mg/kg IV q24h OR penicillin 300,000 U/kg/day IV div q4h; either for 14–28 days
Erythema migrans	Oral therapy as outlined above; for 21 days (AIII)	
Isolated facial (Bell) palsy	Oral therapy as outlined above; for 21–28 days (AIII)	LP is not routinely required unless CNS symptoms present
Carditis	Ceftriaxone 75–100 mg/kg IV q24h OR penicillin 300,000 U/kg/day IV div q4h for 14–28 days (AIII)	
Neuroborreliosis	Ceftriaxone 75–100 mg/kg IV q24h, or penicillin G 300,000 U/kg/day IV div q4h for 14–28 days (AIII)	
Melioidosis (Burkholderia pseudomallei)	Acute sepsis: meropenem 60 mg/kg/day div q8h; OR ceftazidime 150 mg/kg/day IV div q8h; followed by TMP/SMX (8 mg/kg/day of TMP) PO div bid for 3–6 mo	Alternative convalescent therapy: amox/clav (90 mg/kg/day amox div tid, not bid) for children ≤7 y, or doxycycline for children >7 y; for 20 wk (AII)

L. MISCELLANEOUS SYSTEMIC INFECTIONS (cont)

Clinical Diagnosis	Therapy (evidence grade)	Comments
Mycobacteria, nontuberculous		
– Adenitis in normal host (see Adenitis under Skin infections)	Excision usually curative (BII); azithromycin PO OR clarithromycin PO for 6–12 wk (with or without rifampin) if susceptible (BII)	Antibiotic susceptibility patterns are quite variable; cultures should guide therapy; medical therapy 60%–70% effective. Newer data suggest toxicity of antimicrobials may not be worth the small clinical benefit.
– Pneumonia or disseminated infection in compromised hosts (HIV or gamma interferon receptor deficiency)	Usually treated with 3 or 4 active drugs (eg, clarithromycin OR azithromycin, AND amikacin, cefoxitin, meropenem). Also test for ciprofloxacin, TMP/SMX, ethambutol, rifampin, linezolid, clofazimine, and doxycycline (BII)	See Chapter 11 for dosages; cultures are essential, as the susceptibility patterns of nontuberculous mycobacteria are varied.
Nocardiosis (*Nocardia asteroides* and *Nocardia brasiliensis*)	TMP/SMX (8 mg/kg/day of TMP) div bid or sulfisoxazole 120–150 mg/kg/day PO div qid for 6–12 wk or longer. For severe infection, particularly in immunocompromised hosts, use ceftriaxone or meropenem AND amikacin 15–20 mg/kg/day IM, IV div q8h (AIII).	Wide spectrum of disease from skin lesions to brain abscess. Surgery when indicated. Alternatives: doxycycline (for children >7 y of age), amox/clav, or linezolid
Plague (*Yersinia pestis*)	Gentamicin 7.5 mg/kg/day IV div q8h (AII)	Doxycycline 4 mg/kg/day (max 200 mg/day) PO div bid; or ciprofloxacin 30 mg/kg/day PO div bid
Q fever (*Coxiella burnetii*)	Acute stage: doxycycline 4 mg/kg/day (max 200 mg/day) PO div bid for 14 days (AII) for children of any age Endocarditis and chronic disease (>12 mo): doxycycline for children >7 y AND hydroxychloroquine for 18–36 mo (AIII); for children ≤7 y: TMP-SMX, 8–10 mg TMP/kg/day div q12h for 18 mo	CNS: Use fluoroquinolone (no prospective data) (BII). Clarithromycin may be an alternative based on limited data (CIII).

Rocky Mountain spotted fever (fever, petechial rash with centripetal spread; *Rickettsia rickettsii*)	Doxycycline 4 mg/kg/day (max 200 mg/day; PO div bid for 7–10 days (AI) for children of any age	Start empiric therapy early.
Tetanus (*Clostridium tetani*)	Metronidazole 30 mg/kg/day IV, PO div q8h or penicillin G 100,000 U/kg/day V div q6h for 10–14 days AND tetanus immune globulin (TIG) 3,000–6,000 U IM (AII)	Wound debridement essential; IVIG may provide antibody to toxin if TIG not available Immunize with Td or Tdap
Toxic shock syndrome (toxin-producing strains of S aureus or group A streptococcus)	Empiric Vancomycin 45 mg/kg/day IV div q8h AND oxacillin/nafcillin 150 mg/kg/day IV d iv q6h, AND clindamycin 30–40 mg/kg/day div q8h ±gentamicin for 7–10 days (AII)	Clindamycin added for the initial 48–72 h of therapy to decrease toxin production; IVIG may be added to bind circulating toxin For MSSA: oxacillin/nafcillin AND clindamycin ±gentamicin For CA-MRSA: vancomycin AND clindamycin ±gentamicin For group A streptococcus: penicillin G AND clindamycin
Tularemia (*Francisella tularensis*)	Gentamicin 6–7.5 mg/kg/day IM, IV div q8h; for 10–14 days (AII)	Alternatives: doxycycline (for 14–21 days) or ciprofloxacin (for 10 days)

7. Preferred Therapy for Specific Bacterial and Mycobacterial Pathogens

NOTES

- For fungal, viral, and parasitic infections see Chapters 8, 9, and 10, respectively.

- Limitations of space do not permit listing of all possible alternative antimicrobials.

- **Abbreviations:** amox/clav, amoxicillin/clavulanate (Augmentin); amp/sul, ampicillin/sulbactam (Unasyn); CA-MRSA, community-associated methicillin-resistant *Staphylococcus aureus;* CDC, Centers for Disease Control and Prevention; CNS, central nervous system; ESBL, extended spectrum beta-lactamase; HRSA, Health Resources and Services Administration; IM, intramuscular; IV, intravenous; KPC, *Klebsiella pneumoniae* carbapenemase; MRSA, methicillin-resistant *S aureus;* MSSA, methicillin-susceptible *S aureus;* pen-S, penicillin-susceptible; pip/tazo, piperacillin/tazobactam (Zosyn); PO, oral; PZA, pyrazinamide; qd, once daily; ticar/clav, ticarcillin/clavulanate (Timentin); TMP/SMX, trimethoprim/sulfamethoxazole; UTI, urinary tract infection.

Organism	Clinical Illness	Drug of Choice (evidence grade)	Alternatives
Acinetobacter baumanii	Sepsis, meningitis, nosocomial pneumonia	Meropenem (BIII) or other carbapenem	Use culture results to guide therapy: ceftazidime, amp/sul; pip/tazo; TMP/SMX; ciprofloxacin; tigecycline; colistin
Actinobacillus (now *Aggregatibacter*) *actinomycetemcomitans*	Abscesses, endocarditis	Ampicillin (amoxicillin) ± gentamicin (CIII)	Doxycycline; TMP/SMX; ciprofloxacin; ceftriaxone
Actinomyces israelii	Actinomycosis (cervicofacial, thoracic, abdominal)	Penicillin G; ampicillin (CIII)	Amoxicillin; doxycycline; clindamycin; ceftriaxone; imipenem
Aeromonas hydrophila	Diarrhea	Ciprofloxacin (CIII)	Azithromycin, cefepime, TMP/SMX
	Sepsis, cellulitis, necrotizing fasciitis	Ceftazidime (BIII)	Cefepime; ceftriaxone, meropenem; ciprofloxacin
Arcanobacterium haemolyticum	Pharyngitis	Erythromycin; penicillin (BIII)	Azithromycin, amoxicillin, clindamycin; doxycycline; vancomycin
Bacillus anthracis	Anthrax	Ciprofloxacin (regardless of age) (AIII)	Doxycycline; amoxicillin, levofloxacin, clindamycin; penicillin G; vancomycin, meropenem
Bacillus cereus or *subtilis*	Sepsis, endophthalmitis; toxin-mediated gastroenteritis	Vancomycin (BIII)	Clindamycin; meropenem, ciprofloxacin
Bacteroides fragilis	Peritonitis, sepsis, abscesses	Metronidazole (AI)	Meropenem or imipenem (AI); ticar/clav; pip/tazo (AI); clindamycin (AI) with recent surveillance suggesting resistance up to 25%; amox/clav (BII)
Bacteroides, other spp	Pneumonia, sepsis, abscesses	Metronidazole (BII); clindamycin (BII)	Meropenem or imipenem; penicillin G or ampicillin if beta-lactamase negative

Bartonella henselae	Cat-scratch disease	Azithromycin for lymph node disease (BII); gentamicin in combination with TMP/SMX AND rifampin for invasive disease (BIII)	Cefotaxime; ciprofloxacin; doxycycline
Bartonella quintana	Bacillary angiomatosis, peliosis hepatis	Gentamicin plus doxycycline (BIII); erythromycin; ciprofloxacin (BIII)	Azithromycin; doxycycline
Bordetella pertussis, parapertussis	Pertussis	Azithromycin (AIII); erythromycin (BII)	Clarithromycin; TMP/SMX; ampicillin
Borrelia burgdorferi, Lyme disease	Treatment based on stage of infection; see Lyme disease in Chapter 4	Doxycycline if >8 y (AII); amoxicillin or erythromycin in children ≤7 y (AIII); ceftriaxone IV for meningitis (AII)	
Borrelia recurrentis, louse-borne relapsing fever	Relapsing fever	Single dose doxycycline if >8 y (AIII); penicillin or erythromycin in children ≤7 y (BIII)	
Borrelia hermsii, turicatae, parkeri, tickborne relapsing fever	Relapsing fever	Doxycycline if >8 y (AIII); penicillin or erythromycin in children ≤7 y (BIII)	
Brucella spp	Brucellosis (see Chapter 6)	Doxycycline AND rifampin (BIII); TMP/SMX AND rifampin (BIII)	For serious infection: doxycycline AND gentamicin; or TMP/SMX AND gentamicin (AIII)
Burkholderia cepacia complex	Pneumonia, sepsis in immunocompromised children; pneumonia in children with cystic fibrosis	Meropenem (BIII); for severe disease, ADD tobramycin AND TMP/SMX (AIII)	TMP/SMX; doxycycline; ceftazidime; ciprofloxacin Aerosolized antibiotics may provide higher concentrations in lung
Burkholderia pseudomallei	Melioidosis	Meropenem (AIII) or ceftazidime (BIII); followed by prolonged TMP/SMX (AIII)	TMP/SMX, doxycycline, or amox/clav for chronic disease
Campylobacter fetus	Sepsis, meningitis in the neonate	Meropenem (BIII)	Cefotaxime; gentamicin; erythromycin

Organism	Clinical Illness	Drug of Choice (evidence grade)	Alternatives
Campylobacter jejuni	Diarrhea	Azithromycin (BIII); erythromycin (BII)	Doxycycline; ciprofloxacin (very high rates of cipro-R strains in Thailand, Hong Kong and Spain)
Capnocytophaga canimorsus	Sepsis after dog bite	Amox/clav (BIII); penicillin G (BIII)	Ceftriaxone; meropenem; ciprofloxacin; clindamycin; pip/tazo
Capnocytophaga ochracea	Sepsis, abscesses	Clindamycin (BIII); amox/clav (BIII)	Meropenem; ciprofloxacin; pip/tazo
Chlamydophila (formerly *Chlamydia*) *pneumoniae*	Pneumonia	Azithromycin (AII); erythromycin (AII)	Doxycycline; ciprofloxacin
Chlamydophila (formerly *Chlamydia*) *psittaci*	Psittacosis	Azithromycin (AIII); erythromycin (AIII	Doxycycline
Chlamydia trachomatis	Lymphogranuloma venereum	Doxycycline (AII)	Azithromycin; erythromycin
	Urethritis, vaginitis	Doxycycline (AII)	Azithromycin; erythromycin; ofloxacin
	Inclusion conjunctivitis of newborn	Azithromycin (AIII)	Erythromycin
	Pneumonia of infancy	Azithromycin (AIII)	Erythromycin; ampicillin
	Trachoma	Azithromycin (AI)	Doxycycline; erythromycin
Chromobacterium violaceum	Sepsis, pneumonia, abscesses	TMP/SMX AND ciprofloxacin (AIII)	Chloramphenicol ± gentamicin, meropenem
Chryseobacterium (Elizabethkingia) meningosepticum	Sepsis, meningitis	Levofloxacin; TMP/SMX (BIII)	Pip/tazo
Citrobacter spp	Meningitis, sepsis	Meropenem (AIII)	Cefepime; ceftriaxone AND gentamicin; TMP/SMX; ciprofloxacin

Clostridium botulinum	Botulism: foodborne; wound	Botulism antitoxin heptavalent (equine) types A-G (H-BAT) is now the only antitoxin available in the US, through CDC, under an investigational protocol. No antibiotic treatment	Investigational equine antitoxin available only through state health departments or by phone through CDC Emergency Operations Center, 770/488-7100 Additional information on botulism at http://www.bt.cdc.gov/agent/botulism/ and information on H-BAT at (http://www.cdc.gov/ncidod/srp/drugs/formulary.html) (accessed 8/31/11)
	Infant botulism	Human botulism immune globulin BabyBIG) (All) No antibiotic treatment	BabyBIG available nationally from the California State Health Dept at 510/231-7600 (www.dhs.ca.gov/ps/dcdc/InfantBot/ibtindex.htm) (accessed 8/31/11)
Clostridium difficile	Antibiotic-associated colitis (see Chapter 6, Gastrointestinal Infections, *C difficile*)	Metronidazole PO (AI)	Vancomycin PO for metronidazole failures; stop the predisposing antimicrobial therapy, if possible No pediatric data on fidaxomicin PO
Clostridium perfringens	Gas gangrene, sepsis Food poisoning	Penicillin G or clindamycin for invasive infection (BII); no antimicrobials indicated for foodborne illness	Meropenem, metronidazole

Organism	Clinical Illness	Drug of Choice (evidence grade)	Alternatives
Clostridium tetani	Tetanus	Metronidazole (AIII); penicillin G (BIII)	ADD tetanus immune globulin for contaminated wounds at 250 U IM for those with <3 tetanus immunizations; for treatment of symptomatic infection: 3,000 to 6,000 U IM, with part injected directly into the wound Alternative antibiotics: meropenem; doxycycline, clindamycin Immunize after recovery.
Corynebacterium diphtheriae	Diphtheria	Diphtheria equine antitoxin (available through CDC, under an investigational protocol) AND erythromycin or penicillin G (AIII)	Antitoxin from the CDC at 404/639-8257 or the Emergency Operations Center 770/488-7100 (http://www.cdc.gov/ncidod/srp/drugs/formulary.html. Accessed 8/31/11)
Corynebacterium jeikeium	Sepsis, endocarditis	Vancomycin (AIII)	Penicillin G AND gentamicin
Corynebacterium minutissimum	Erythrasma; bacteremia in compromised hosts	Erythromycin PO for erythrasma (BIII); vancomycin IV for bacteremia (BIII)	Topical clindamycin for cutaneous infection
Coxiella burnetii	Q fever	Doxycycline (all ages) (AII)	Ciprofloxacin
Ehrlichia chafeensis	Human monocytic ehrlichiosis	Doxycycline (all ages) (AII)	Rifampin
E ewingii	*E ewingii* ehrlichiosis	Doxycycline (all ages) (AII)	Rifampin
Ehrlichia (now *Anaplasma*) *phagocytophilum*	Human granulocytic anaplasmosis	Doxycycline (all ages) (AII)	Rifampin
Eikenella corrodens	Human bite wounds; abscesses, meningitis	Ampicillin; penicillin G (BIII)	Amox/clav; ticar/clav; pip/tazo; amp/sul; ceftriaxone; ciprofloxacin Resistant to clindamycin, cephalexin, erythromycin

Organism	Condition		
Enterobacter spp	Sepsis, pneumonia, wound infection, UTI	Cefepime; meropenem (BII)	Ertapenem; imipenem; cefotaxime or ceftriaxone AND gentamicin; TMP/SMX; ciprofloxacin Newly emerging carbapenem-R strains worldwide
Enterococcus spp	Endocarditis UTI	Ampicillin AND gentamicin (AI)	Vancomycin AND gentamicin For vancomycin-resistant strains that are also amp-R: linezolid, daptomycin, tigecycline
Erysipelothrix rhusiopathiae	Sepsis, cellulitis, abscesses, endocarditis	Ampicillin (BIII); penicillin G (BIII)	Ceftriaxone; clindamycin, meropenem; ciprofloxacin Resistant to vancomycin, daptomycin, TMP/SMX
Escherichia coli See Chapter 6 for specific infection entities with *E coli*.	UTI, not hospital-acquired	A 2nd or 3rd generation cephalosporin PO, IM (BI)	Amoxicillin; TMP/SMX if susceptible For hospital-acquired UTI, review hospital antibiogram for choices.
	Traveler's diarrhea	Azithromycin (AII)	Rifaximin (for nonfebrile, nonbloody diarrhea for children >11 y); cefixime
	Sepsis, pneumonia, hospital-acquired UTI	A 2nd or 3rd generation cephalosporin IV (BI)	For ESBL-producing strains: meropenem (AIII) or other carbapenem
			Ciprofloxacin if resistant to other antibiotics
	Meningitis	Ceftriaxone; cefotaxime (AIII)	For ESBL-producing strains: meropenem (AIII)
Francisella tularensis	Tularemia	Gentamicin (AII)	Doxycycline; ciprofloxacin
Fusobacterium spp	Sepsis, soft tissue infection, Lemierre syndrome	Metronidazole (AIII); clindamycin (BIII)	Penicillin G; meropenem

Organism	Clinical Illness	Drug of Choice (evidence grade)	Alternatives
Gardnerella vaginalis	Bacterial vaginosis	Metronidazole (BII)	Clindamycin
Haemophilus aphrophilus	Sepsis, endocarditis, abscesses	Ceftriaxone (AII); OR ampicillin AND gentamicin (BII)	Ciprofloxacin, amox/clav
Haemophilus ducreyi	Chancroid	Azithromycin (AIII); ceftriaxone (BIII)	Erythromycin; ciprofloxacin
Haemophilus influenzae			
– Non-encapsulated strains	Upper respiratory tract infections	Beta-lactamase neg: ampicillin IV (AI); amoxicillin PO (AI)	Levofloxacin; azithromycin; TMP/SMX
– Type b strains	Meningitis, arthritis, cellulitis, epiglottitis, pneumonia	Beta-lactamase positive: ceftriaxone IV, IM (AI), or cefotaxime IV (AI); amox/clav (AI) OR 2nd or 3rd generation cephalosporins PO (AI)	Full IV course (10 days) for meningitis
Helicobacter pylori	Gastritis, peptic ulcer	Clarithromycin AND amoxicillin AND omeprazole (AII)	Other regimens include metronidazole (especially for concerns of clarithro-R), and other proton pump inhibitors
Klebsiella spp (*K pneumoniae*, *K oxytoca*)	UTI	A 2nd or 3rd generation cephalosporin (AII)	Use most narrow spectrum agent active against pathogen: TMP/SMX; gentamicin ESBL producers should be treated with a carbapenem (meropenem, ertapenem, imipenem), but KPC-containing carbapenem-R organisms may require colistin
	Sepsis, pneumonia, meningitis	Ceftriaxone; cefotaxime, cefepime (AIII)	Carbapenem or ciprofloxacin if resistant to other routine antibiotics Meningitis caused by ESBL producer: meropenem KPC carbapenemase producers: ciprofloxacin, colistin

Klebsiella granulomatis	Granuloma inguinale	Doxycycline (AII)	Azithromycin; TMP/SMX; ciprofloxacin
Kingella kingae	Osteomyelitis, arthritis	Ampicillin; penicillin G (AII)	Ceftriaxone; TMP/SMX; oxacillin/ nafcillin; cephalexin; ciprofloxacin
Legionella spp	Legionnaires disease	Azithromycin (AI)	Erythromycin; levofloxacin; doxycycline
Leptospira spp	Leptospirosis	Penicillin G(AII); ceftriaxone(AII)	Amoxicillin; doxycycline
Leuconostoc	Bacteremia	Penicillin G (AIII); ampicillin (BIII)	Clindamycin; erythromycin; doxycycline (resistant to vancomycin)
Listeria monocytogenes	Sepsis, meningitis in compromised host; neonatal sepsis	Ampicillin (ADD gentamicin for severe infection) (AII)	TMP/SMX; vancomycin
Moraxella catarrhalis	Otitis, sinusitis, bronchitis	Amox/clav (AI)	TMP/SMX; a 2nd or 3rd generation cephalosporin
Morganella morganii	UTI, sepsis, wound infection	Cefepime (AIII); meropenem (AIII)	Pip/tazo; ceftriaxone AND gentamicin
Mycobacterium abscessus	Skin and soft tissue infections; pneumonia in cystic fibrosis	Clarithromycin or azithromycin (AIII); ADD amikacin ± cefoxitin for invasive disease (AIII)	Also test for susceptibility to: tigecycline, linezolid
Mycobacterium avium complex	Cervical adenitis, pneumonia	Clarithromycin (AII); azithromycin (AI)	Surgical excision may be curative. May increase cure rate with addition of rifampin ± ethambutol.
	Disseminated disease in competent host, or disease in immunocompromised host	Clarithromycin or azithromycin AND ethambutol AND rifampin (AIII)	Depending on susceptibilities, and the severity of illness, ADD amikacin ± ciprofloxacin.
Mycobacterium bovis	Tuberculosis (adenitis; abdominal tuberculosis meningitis)	Isoniazid AND rifampin (AII); add ethambutol for suspected resistance (AII)	Add streptomycin for severe infection.
			M bovis is resistant to PZA.

Organism	Clinical Illness	Drug of Choice (evidence grade)	Alternatives
Mycobacterium chelonae	Abscesses; catheter infection	Clarithromycin or azithromycin (AIII); ADD amikacin ± cefoxitin for invasive disease (AIII)	Also test for susceptibility to cefoxitin; TMP/SMX; doxycycline; gentamicin, imipenem; moxifloxacin, linezolid.
Mycobacterium fortuitum complex	Skin and soft tissue infections; catheter infection	Amikacin AND imipenem (AIII) ± ciprofloxacin (AIII)	Also test for susceptibility to cefoxitin; sulfonamides; doxycycline; linezolid.
Mycobacterium leprae	Leprosy	Dapsone AND rifampin (for pauci-bacillary) (AII) ADD clarithromycin for lepromatous, multibacillary disease (AII)	Consult HRSA (National Hansen's Disease Program) at http://www.hrsa.gov/hansensdisease/ for advice about treatment and free antibiotics: 800/642-2477.
Mycobacterium marinum/balnei	Papules, pustules, abscesses (swimmer's granuloma)	Clarithromycin ± rifampin (AIII)	TMP/SMX AND rifampin; doxycycline; ethambutol
Mycobacterium tuberculosis	Tuberculosis (pneumonia; meningitis; cervical adenitis; mesenteric adenitis; osteomyelitis)	Isoniazid AND rifampin AND PZA (AI)	Add ethambutol for suspect resistance; add streptomycin for severe infection. Corticosteroids should be added to regimens for meningitis, mesenteric adenitis, and endobronchial infection (AIII).
Mycoplasma hominis	Non-gonococcal urethritis; neonatal infection	Clindamycin (AIII)	Fluoroquinolones; doxycycline Usually erythromycin-resistant
Mycoplasma pneumoniae	Pneumonia	Azithromycin (AI); erythromycin (BI)	Doxycycline; fluoroquinolones
Neisseria gonorrhoeae	Gonorrhea; arthritis	Ceftriaxone (AI); cefixime (AI)	Spectinomycin IM

		Ceftriaxone (AI); cefotaxime (AI)	Penicillin G or ampicillin
Neisseria meningitidis	Sepsis, meningitis		For prophylaxis following exposure: rifampin or ciprofloxacin (ciprofloxacin-resistant strains have now been reported)
Nocardia asteroides or *brasiliensis*	Nocardiosis	TMP/SMX (AII); sulfisoxazole (BII); (AND amikacin for severe infection) (AII)	Meropenem; ceftriaxone; doxycycline; linezolid
Oerskovic (now known as *Cellulosimicrobium cellulans*)	Wound infection; catheter infection	Vancomycin ± rifampin (AIII)	Resistant to beta-lactams, macrolides, aminoglycosides
Pasteurella multocida	Sepsis, abscesses, animal bite wound	Penicillin G (AIII); ampicillin (AIII); amoxicillin (AIII)	Amox/clav; ticar/clav; pip/tazo; doxycycline; ceftriaxone
Peptostreptococcus	Sepsis, deep head/neck space and intra-abdominal infection	Penicillin G (AIII); ampicillin (AII)	Clindamycin; vancomycin; meropenem/ imipenem, metronidazole
Plesiomonas shigelloides	Diarrhea, meningitis	Antibiotics may not be necessary to treat diarrhea; 2nd and 3rd generation cephalosporins (AIII); azithromycin (BIII); ciprofloxacin (CIII)	For meningitis/sepsis: meropenem; pip/tazo; ceftriaxone
Prevotella (Bacteroides) melaninogenicus	Deep head/neck space abscess; dental abscess	Metronidazole (AII); meropenem/ imipenem (AII)	Pip/tazo; clindamycin
Propionibacterium acnes	In addition to acne, invasive infection; sepsis, postop wound infection	Penicillin (AIII); vancomycin (AIII) wound infection	Cefotaxime; doxycycline; clindamycin; ciprofloxacin; linezolid
Proteus mirabilis	UTI, sepsis, meningitis	Ampicillin (AII)	Increasing resistance, particularly in nosocomial isolates. Use most narrow spectrum agent active against pathogen; TMP/SMX; a cephalosporin; an aminoglycoside.

Organism	Clinical Illness	Drug of Choice (evidence grade)	Alternatives
Proteus vulgaris, other spp (indole-positive strains)	UTI, sepsis, meningitis	Ceftriaxone (AII); cefotaxime (AII)	Cefepime; meropenem; gentamicin; ciprofloxacin; TMP/SMX
Providencia spp	Sepsis	Ceftriaxone (AII); cefotaxime (AII)	Cefepime; meropenem; gentamicin; ciprofloxacin; TMP/SMX
Pseudomonas aeruginosa	UTI	Ceftazidime (AII); other anti-pseudomonal beta-lactams	Tobramycin; amikacin; ciprofloxacin
	Nosocomial sepsis, pneumonia	Cefepime (AI) or meropenem (AI); OR ceftazidime AND tobramycin (BI)	Pip/tazo AND tobramycin (BI); ciprofloxacin AND tobramycin
	Pneumonia in cystic fibrosis	Cefepime (AII) or meropenem (AII); OR ceftazidime AND tobramycin (BII); ADD aerosol tobramycin (AI) Azithromycin appears to provide benefit from anti-inflammatory properties.	Insufficient data to yet recommend aztreonam aerosol Many organisms are multidrug resistant; consider ciprofloxacin or colistin parenterally; in vitro synergy testing may suggest effective combinations. For multidrug-resistant organisms, colistin aerosol (AIII)
Pseudomonas cepacia, mallei, or pseudomallei (see *Burkholderia*)			
Rhodococcus equi	Necrotizing pneumonia	Imipenem AND vancomycin (AIII)	Amikacin; erythromycin; rifampin; ciprofloxacin
Rickettsia	Rocky Mountain spotted fever, Q fever, typhus, rickettsial pox	Doxycycline (all ages) (AII)	Chloramphenicol; a fluoroquinolone
Salmonella, non-typhi	Gastroenteritis; focal infections; bacteremia	Ceftriaxone (AII); cefixime (AII); azithromycin (AII)	For susceptible strains: ciprofloxacin; TMP/SMX; ampicillin
Salmonella typhi	Typhoid fever	Ceftriaxone (AII); azithromycin (AII); ciprofloxacin (AII)	For susceptible strains: TMP/SMX; ampicillin

Organism	Infection	Treatment	Alternative
Serratia marcescens	Nosocomial sepsis, pneumonia	Cefepime (AII); a carbapenem (AII)	Ceftriaxone or cefotaxime AND gentamicin; or ciprofloxacin
Shigella spp	Enteritis, UTI, prepubertal vaginitis	Ceftriaxone (AII); azithromycin (AIII); cefixime (AII); ciprofloxacin (AII)	Use most narrow spectrum agent active against pathogen: ampicillin (not amoxicillin); TMP/SMX
Spirillum minus	Rat-bite fever (sodoku fever)	Pen icillin G V (AIII); for endocarditis, ADD gentamicin or streptomycin (AIII)	Ampicillin; doxycycline; cefotaxime, vancomycin, streptomycin
Staphylococcus aureus (see Chapter 4: CA-MRSA)			
Mild-moderate infections	Skin infections, mild–moderate	MSSA: a 1st generation cephalosporin (cefazolin IV, cephalexin PO) (AI); oxacillin/nafcillin IV (AI), dicloxacillin PO (AI) MRSA: vancomycin IV or clindamycin IV or PO (AIII)	For MSSA: amox/clav For CA-MRSA: TMP/SMX (if susceptible); linezolid IV, PO; daptomycin IV
Moderate-severe infections, treat empirically for CA-MRSA	Pneumonia, sepsis, myositis, osteomyelitis, etc	MSSA: oxacillin/nafcillin IV (AI); a 1st generation cephalosporin (cefazolin IV) (AI) ± gentamicin (AIII) MRSA: vancomycin (AII) or clindamycin (AIII); ± gentamicin ± rifampin (AIII)	For CA-MRSA: linezolid (AII); OR daptomycin for non-pulmonary infection (AII) Insufficient data to recommend ceftaroline in pediatrics
Staphylococcus, coagulase negative	Nosocomial sepsis, infected CNS shunts, UTI	Vancomycin (AII)	If susceptible: nafcillin (or other anti-staph beta-lactam); rifampin (in combination); linezolid
Stenotrophomonas maltophilia	Sepsis	TMP/SMX (AII)	Ceftazidime; ticar/clav; doxycycline; levofloxacin
Streptobacillus moniliformis	Rat-bite fever (Haverhill fever)	Penicillin G (AIII); ampicillin (AIII); for endocarditis, ADD gentamicin or streptomycin (AIII)	Doxycycline; ceftriaxone; carbapenems; clindamycin; vancomycin

Organism	Clinical Illness	Drug of Choice (evidence grade)	Alternatives
Streptococcus, group A	Pharyngitis, impetigo, adenitis, cellulitis, necrotizing fasciitis	Penicillin (AI); amoxicillin (AI)	A 1st generation cephalosporin (cefazolin, or cephalexin) (AI); clindamycin (AI); a macrolide (AI), vancomycin (AIII) For relapsing pharyngitis, clindamycin or amox/clav (AIII)
Streptococcus, group B	Neonatal sepsis, pneumonia, meningitis	Penicillin (AII) or ampicillin (AII) ± gentamicin (AIII)	Vancomycin (AIII)
Streptococcus, milleri/anginosus group (*S intermedius, anginosus,* and *constellatus*; includes some beta-hemolytic group C and group G streptococci)	Pneumonia, sepsis, skin and soft tissue infection, sinusitis, arthritis, brain abscess, meningitis	Penicillin G (AIII); ampicillin (AIII) ADD gentamicin for serious infection (AIII). Many strains may show decreased susceptibility to penicillin.	Clindamycin; a 1st generation cephalosporin; vancomycin
Streptococcus pneumoniae With widespread use of conjugate pneumococcal vaccines, antibiotic resistance in pneumococci has decreased substantially.	Otitis, sinusitis	Amoxicillin, high-dose (90 mg/kg/day) (AII)	Amox/clav; cefdinir; cefpodoxime; cefuroxime; azithromycin; clarithromycin; OR ceftriaxone IM
	Meningitis	Ceftriaxone (AI) or cefotaxime (AII); AND vancomycin for possible ceftriaxone-resistant strains (AIII)	Penicillin G alone for pen-S strains; ceftriaxone alone for ceftriaxone-susceptible strains
	Pneumonia, osteomyelitis/arthritis, sepsis	Ampicillin (AII); ceftriaxone (AI); cefotaxime (AI)	Penicillin G for pen-S strains (AI)

Organism	Clinical condition		
Streptococcus, viridans group (alpha-hemolytic streptococci, most commonly S sanguis, S oralis (mitis), S salivarius, S mutans, S mortillorum)	Endocarditis	Penicillin G ± gentamicin (AII) OR ceftriaxone ± gentamicin (AII)	Vancomycin
Treponema pallidum	Syphilis	Penicillin G (AII)	Doxycycline; ceftriaxone
Ureaplasma urealyticum	Genitourinary infections; Neonatal pneumonia (therapy may not be effective)	Azithromycin (AII); Azithromycin (AIII)	Erythromycin; doxycycline, ofloxacin (for adolescent genital infections)
Vibrio cholerae	Cholera	Doxycycline (AI) or azithromycin (AII)	Ciprofloxacin; TMP/SMX
Vibrio vulnificus	Sepsis, necrotizing fasciitis	Doxycycline AND ceftazidime (AIII)	Ciprofloxacin AND cefotaxime
Yersinia enterocolitica	Diarrhea, mesenteric enteritis, reactive arthritis, sepsis	TMP/SMX (AIII); ciprofloxacin (AIII)	Ceftriaxone; gentamicin
Yersinia pestis	Plague	Gentamicin (AIII)	Doxycycline; ciprofloxacin
Yersinia pseudotuberculosis	Mesenteric adenitis; Far East scarlet fever; reactive arthritis	TMP/SMX (AIII); ciprofloxacin (AIII)	Ceftriaxone; gentamicin

8. Preferred Therapy for Specific Fungal Pathogens

NOTES

- See Chapter 2 for discussion of polyenes, azoles, and echinocandins.

- **Abbreviations:** AmB-D, amphotericin B deoxycholate, the oldest, standard AmB (original trade name Fungizone); ABLC, amphotericin B lipid complex (Abelcet); ABCD, amphotericin B colloidal suspension (Amphotec); bid, twice daily; CNS, central nervous system; CSF, cerebrospinal fluid; div, divided; L-AmB, liposomal amphotericin B (AmBisome); IV, intravenous; PO, orally; qd, once daily; qid, 4 times daily; soln, solution; tab, tablet; tid, 3 times daily; TMP/SMX, trimethoprim/sulfamethoxazole.

A. SYSTEMIC INFECTIONS

Infection	Therapy (evidence grade)	Comments
PROPHYLAXIS		
Prophylaxis of invasive fungal infection in patients with hematologic malignancies	Fluconazole 6 mg/kg/day for prevention of *Candida* infection (AII)	Fluconazole is not effective against *Aspergillus* and some strains of *Candida*. Posaconazole PO, voriconazole PO, and micafungin IV are effective in adults in preventing *Aspergillus* and *Candida* but are not well studied in children, and should only be used for highest risk patients.
Prophylaxis of invasive fungal infection in patients with solid organ transplants	Fluconazole 6 mg/kg/day for prevention of *Candida* infection (AII)	AmB, caspofungin, micafungin, voriconazole, or posaconazole may be effective in preventing *Aspergillus* infection.
TREATMENT		
Aspergillosis	Voriconazole 18 mg/kg/day IV div q12h for a loading dose on the first day, then 16 mg/kg/day IV div q12h as a maintenance dose for children 2–12 y. In children >12 y, use adult dosing (load 12 mg/kg/day IV div q12h on first day, then 8 mg/kg/day div q12h as a maintenance dose) (AII). When stable, may switch from voriconazole IV to voriconazole PO at a dose of 18 mg/kg/day div bid for children 2–12 y and 400 mg/day div bid for children >12 y (AIII). Alternatives: Caspofungin 70 mg/m² IV loading dose on day 1 (max dose 70 mg), followed by 50 mg/m² IV (max dose 70 mg) on subsequent days (BII) OR L-AmB 3–5 mg/kg/day as 3–4 h infusions (in adults, higher dosages have not produced improved outcome) (AII).	Voriconazole is the preferred primary antifungal therapy for all clinical forms of *Aspergillus* infection. Optimal voriconazole trough serum concentrations (generally thought to be >1–2 µg/mL) are important for success. Total treatment course is at least 6 wk or until disease controlled. Salvage therapy options include a change of antifungal class (using L-AmB or an echinocandin), switching to posaconazole, or using combination antifungal therapy. Combination therapy is not well studied prospectively in controlled clinical trials. In vitro data suggest greatest synergy with 2 (but not 3) drug combinations: an azole plus an echinocandin is the most well studied. Both voriconazole and AmB are fungicidal, while the echinocandins are fungistatic. *Aspergillus terreus* is AmB-resistant.

		Against most *Aspergillus* sp, micafungin demonstrates equivalent activity to caspofungin. Immune reconstitution is paramount to treatment success; for children receiving corticosteroids, decreasing the corticosteroid dosage is also important.
Blastomycosis (North American)	For moderate to severe disease: ABLC or L-AmB 3–5 mg/kg IV daily as 3–4 h infusion for 1–2 wk or until improvement noted, followed by oral itraconazole 10 mg/kg/day div bid (max 600 mg/day) PO for a total of 12 mo (AIII) For mild-moderate disease: oral itraconazole 10 mg/kg/day div bid (max 600 mg/day) PO for a total of 6–12 mo (AIII)	Itraconazole oral soln provides greater and more reliable absorption than capsules; serum concentrations of itraconazole should be determined 2 wk after start of therapy to ensure adequate drug exposure (maintain trough levels >0.5 μg/mL). Alternative: high-dose fluconazole (BIII), especially useful in CNS disease. Patients with extrapulmonary blastomycosis should receive at least 12 mo of total therapy. CNS blastomycosis should begin with ABLC/L-AmB for 4–6 wk, followed by an azole for a total therapy of at least 12 mo until resolution of CSF abnormalities. Lifelong itraconazole if immunosuppression cannot be reversed.

A. SYSTEMIC INFECTIONS (cont)

Infection	Therapy (evidence grade)	Comments
Candidiasis (see Chapter 2) – Disseminated infection	For neutropenic patients: An echinocandin is recommended. Caspofungin 70 mg/m² IV loading dose on day 1 (max dose 70 mg), followed by 50 mg/m² IV (max dose 70 mg) on subsequent days (AII); OR micafungin 2–4 mg/kg/day q24h for children ≤40 kg, and 100 mg/day q24h for children >40 kg (BIII); preterm neonates may require up to 10–15 mg/kg/day to achieve adequate drug exposure (BIII) OR ABLC or L-AmB 5 mg/kg/day IV q24h (BII). For neutropenic but less critically ill patients with no recent azole exposure, fluconazole (12 mg/kg/day) is an alternative. For non-neutropenic patients: Fluconazole (12 mg/kg/day) is recommended in those patients who are less critically ill and with no recent azole exposure. An echinocandin is recommended in those non-neutropenic patients who are more critically ill or patients who have had recent azole exposure. L-AmB or ABLC (3–5 mg/kg/day) are alternatives, and voriconazole could be used for step-down oral therapy for C krusei or voriconazole-susceptible C glabrata but otherwise offers little advantage over fluconazole. For CNS infections: AmB-D 1 mg/kg/day or L-AmB/ABLC (3–5 mg/kg/day) AND flucytosine 100 mg/kg/day PO div q6h (AII) until initial clinical response, followed by step-down therapy with fluconazole (12 mg/kg/day); echinocandins do NOT achieve therapeutic concentrations in CSF.	Removal of infected intravenous catheter or any infected devices is critical to success. For infections with C glabrata, an echinocandin is preferred. Transition to an azole as step-down therapy only after confirmation of isolate susceptibility. Patients already receiving an empiric azole who are clinically improving can remain on the azole. For infections with C parapsilosis, fluconazole or ABLC/L-AmB is preferred. Patients already receiving an empiric echinocandin who are clinically improving can remain on the echinocandin. Therapy is for 2 wk after documented clearance in pediatric patients, but 3 wk in neonates due to higher rate of meningitis and dissemination.

– Oropharyngeal, esophageal	Oropharyngeal: Mild disease; clotrimazole 10 mg troches PO 5 times daily OR nystatin (either 100,000 U/mL with 4–6 mL 4 times daily or 1–2 200,000 U pastilles 4 times daily for 7–14 days. Moderate-severe disease: Fluconazole 3–6 mg/kg once daily PO for 7–14 days (AII). Esophageal: Oral fluconazole (6–12 mg/kg/day) for 14–21 days. If cannot tolerate oral therapy, then use fluconazole IV OR ABLC/L-AmB OR an echinocandin.	For fluconazole-refractory disease: Itraconazole OR posaconazole OR AmB IV OR an echinocandin for 14–28 days. Esophageal disease always requires systemic antifungal therapy. Suppressive therapy (3 times weekly) with fluconazole is recommended for recurrent infections.
– Neonatal candidiasis	L-AmB/ABLC (5 mg/kg/day) or AmB-D (1 mg/kg/day). Theoretical risk of AmB-D less penetration, so some would NOT recommend lipid formulation if urinary tract involvement is possible. Fluconazole (12 mg/kg/day, after loading dose of 25 mg/kg) is an alternative (BII). Therapy is for 3 wk (not 2 wk as in pediatric patients).	Nurseries with high rates of candidiasis should consider fluconazole prophylaxis (AI) (3 mg/kg or 6 mg/kg twice weekly) in high-risk neonates (birth weight <1,000 g). Lumbar puncture and thorough retinal examination recommended (BIII). Imaging of genitourinary tract, liver, and spleen recommended if persistently positive cultures (BIII). Assume meningoencephalitis in the neonate due to the high incidence of this complication. Role of flucytosine in neonates with Candida meningitis is questionable and not routinely recommended due to toxicity concerns. Echinocandins are under study and generally used in cases of antifungal resistance or toxicity.
– Peritonitis (secondary to peritoneal dialysis)	Fluconazole 200 mg intraperitoneal q24h (AII)	Remove peritoneal dialysis catheter; replace after 4–6 wk of treatment, if possible. High-dosage oral fluconazole may also be used. AmB should not be instilled into the peritoneal cavity.

A. SYSTEMIC INFECTIONS (cont)

Infection	Therapy (evidence grade)	Comments
– Urinary tract infection	Cystitis: Fluconazole 3–6 mg/kg once daily IV or PO for 2 wk (AIII) Pyelonephritis: Fluconazole 3–6 mg/kg once daily IV or PO for 2 wk (AII)	Removing Foley catheter, if present, may lead to a spontaneous cure in the normal host; check for additional upper urinary tract disease. For fluconazole-resistant organisms, AmB-D is an alternative. AmB-D bladder irrigation is not generally recommended due to high relapse rate (an exception may be in fluconazole-resistant C glabrata or C krusei). For renal collecting system fungus balls, surgical debridement may be required in non-neonates (BIII). Echinocandins have poor urinary concentrations.
– Vulvovaginal	Topical vaginal cream/tabs/suppositories (alphabetic order): Butoconazole, clotrimazole, econazole, fenticonazole, miconazole, sertaconazole, terconazole, or tioconazole for 3–7 days OR Fluconazole 10 mg/kg (max 150 mg) as a single dose (AII)	No topical agent is clearly superior. Avoid azoles during pregnancy. For recurring disease, consider 10–14 days of induction with topical or systemic azole followed by fluconazole once weekly for 6 mo.
– Cutaneous candidiasis	Topical therapy (alphabetic order): Ciclopirox, clotrimazole, econazole, haloprogin, ketoconazole, miconazole, oxiconazole, sertaconazole, sulconazole	Fluconazole 3–6 mg/kg/day PO once daily for 5–7 days
– Chronic mucocutaneous	Fluconazole 3–5 mg/kg daily PO until lesions clear (AII)	Alternative: Itraconazole 5 mg/kg PO soln q24h Relapse common
Chromoblastomycosis	Itraconazole oral soln 10 mg/kg/day div bid PO for 12–18 mo, in combination with surgical excision or repeated cryotherapy (AIII)	Alternative: Terbinafine or an AmB

Coccidioidomycosis	For moderate infections: Fluconazole 12 mg/kg IV, PO q24h (AII) For severe pulmonary disease: AmB-D 1 mg/kg/day IV q24h; OR ABLC or L-AmB 5 mg/kg/day IV q24h (AIII) as initial therapy until clear improvement, followed by an oral azole for total therapy of up to 12 mo, depending on genetic or immunocompromising risk factors. For meningitis: Fluconazole 12 mg/kg/day IV q24h (AII); for failures, intrathecal AmB-D (0.1–1.5 mg/dose) OR voriconazole IV (AIII). Lifelong azole suppressive therapy may be required. For extrapulmonary (nonmeningeal), particularly for osteomyelitis: Itraconazole scln 10 mg/kg/day div bid for 12 mo appears more effective than fluconazole (AIII), and AmB as an alternative if worsening.	Mild pulmonary disease does not require therapy in the normal host and only requires periodic reassessment. Posaconazole also active, but little experience in children. Treat until serum cocci complement fixation titers drop to 1:8 or 1:4, about 3–6 mo. Disease in immunocompromised hosts may need to be treated longer, including potentially lifelong azole secondary prophylaxis. Watch for relapse up to 1–2 y after therapy.
Cryptococcosis	For mild-moderate pulmonary disease: Fluconazole 12 mg/kg/day IV, PO q24h for 6–12 mo (AII) For meningitis or severe pulmonary disease: Incuction therapy with AmB-D 0.7–1.0 mg/kg/day IV q24h OR ABLC or L-AmB 3–5 mg/kg/day q24h; AND flucytosine 100 mg/kg/day PO div q6h for a minimum of 2 wk until CSF cleared, FOLLOWED BY consolidation therapy with fluconazole (12 mg/kg/day) for a minimum of 8 wk (AI).	Monitor flucytosine serum trough concentrations to keep peaks less than 80–100 (and ideally 40–80) μg/mL to prevent neutropenia. For HIV-positive patients, continue maintenance therapy with fluconazole (4 mg/kg/day) indefinitely. In organ transplant recipients, continue maintenance fluconazole (4 mg/kg/day) for 6–12 mo after consolidation therapy. For cryptococcal relapse, restart induction therapy and determine susceptibility of relapse isolate.

A. SYSTEMIC INFECTIONS (cont)

Infection	Therapy (evidence grade)	Comments
Fusarium, Scedosporium prolificans, and **Pseudallescheria boydii** (and its asexual form, **Scedosporium apiospermum**)	Voriconazole 18 mg/kg/day IV div q12h for a loading dose on the first day, then 16 mg/kg/day IV div q12h as a maintenance dose for children 2–12 y. In children >12 y, use adult dosing (load 12 mg/kg/day IV div q12h on first day, then 8 mg/kg/day IV div q12h as a maintenance dose) (AII). When stable, may switch from voriconazole IV to voriconazole PO at a dose of 18 mg/kg/day div bid for children 2–12 y and 400 mg/day div bid for children >12 y (AIII).	Optimal voriconazole trough concentrations (generally thought to be >1–2 μg/mL) are important. Resistant to AmB in vitro. Alternatives: Echinocandins have been successful at salvage therapy anecdotally; posaconazole likely helpful; while there are reports of combinations with terbinafine, terbinafine does not obtain good tissue concentrations for these disseminated infections.
Histoplasmosis	For severe pulmonary disease: AmB-D 1 mg/kg/day q24h OR ABLC/L-AmB at 3–5 mg/kg/day q24h for 1–2 wk, FOLLOWED BY itraconazole 10 mg/kg/day div bid to complete a total of 12 wk (AIII). For mild-moderate acute pulmonary disease, itraconazole 10 mg/kg/day PO soln div BID for 6–12 wk (AIII).	Mild disease may not require therapy and in most cases resolves in 1 mo. For disease with respiratory distress, ADD corticosteroids in first 1–2 wk of antifungal therapy. Progressive disseminated or CNS disease requires AmB therapy for the initial 4–6 wk. Potential lifelong suppressive itraconazole if cannot reverse immunosuppression.
Paracoccidioidomycosis	Itraconazole 10 mg/kg/day PO soln div bid for 6 mo (AIII) OR ketoconazole 5 mg/kg/day PO q24h for 6 mo (BIII).	Alternatives: voriconazole; sulfadiazine or TMP/SMX for 3–5 y. AmB is another alternative and may be combined with sulfa or azole antifungals.
Phaeohyphomycosis (dematiaceous, pigmented fungi)	Voriconazole 18 mg/kg/day IV div q12h for a loading dose on the first day, then 16 mg/kg/day IV div q12h as a maintenance dose for children 2–12 y. In children >12 y, use adult dosing (load 12 mg/kg/day IV div q12h on first day, then 8 mg/kg/day IV div q12h as a maintenance dose) (AII).	Surgery is essential; susceptibilities are variable. Optimal voriconazole trough concentrations (generally thought to be >1–2 μg/mL) are important.

	When stable, may switch from voriconazole IV to voriconazole PO at a dose of 18 mg/kg/day div bid for children 2–12 y and 400 mg/day div bid for children >12 y (AIII). Alternatives could include combination therapy with an echinocandin and an azole, an echinocandin and AmB (AII).	If no response for cutaneous disease, treat with higher itraconazole dose, terbinafine, or saturated soln of potassium iodide. Fluconazole is less effective. Obtain serum concentrations of itraconazole after 2 wk of therapy, want serum trough level >0.5 μ/mL. For meningeal disease, initial AmB should be 4–6 wk before change to itraconazole for a total of 12 mo of therapy. Surgery may be necessary in osteoarticular or pulmonary disease.
Pneumocystis jiroveci (carinii) pneumonia	Serious disease: preferred regimen is TMP/SMX 15–20 mg, TMP/kg/day IV div q6h (AI) for TMP/SMX intolerant or TMP/SMX treatment failure, pentamidine isethionate 4 mg base/kg/day IV daily (BII) ; for 3 wk Mild-moderate disease: start with IV therapy, then after acute pneumonitis is resolved, TMP/SMX, 20 mg TMP/kg/day PO div qid for 3 wk total treatment course (AII)	Alternatives: TMP AND dapsone; OR primaquine AND clindamycin; OR atovaquone Prophylaxis: preferred regimen is TMP/SMX (5 mg TMP component/kg/day) PO div bid, 3x/wk on consecutive days ; OR same dose, given once daily, 3x/wk on consecutive days; OR dapsone 2 mg/kg (max 100 mg) PO once daily, OR dapsone 4 mg/kg (max 200 mg) PO once weekly. Use steroid therapy for more severe disease.
Sporotrichosis	For cutaneous/lymphocutaneous: itraconazole 10 mg/kg/day div bid PO soln for 2–4 wk after all lesions gone (generally total of 3–6 mo) (AII). For serious pulmonary or disseminated infection or disseminated sporotrichosis: ABLC/L-AmB at 3–5 mg/kg/day q24h until stable, then step-down therapy with itraconazole PO for a total of 12 mo (AIII). For less severe disease, itraconazole for 12 mo.	
Zygomycosis (mucormycosis)	Requires aggressive surgery and combination antifungal therapy: ABLC/L-AmB at 5 mg/kg/day q24h AND caspofungin for 6–12 wk or longer (AIII). For AmB failures, posaconazole may be effective against most strains (AIII).	Following clinical response with AmB, long-term oral step-down therapy with posaconazole can be attempted for 2–6 mo. Voriconazole has NO activity against zygomycetes.

B. LOCALIZED MUCOCUTANEOUS INFECTIONS

Infection	Therapy (evidence grade)	Comments
Dermatophytoses		
– Scalp (tinea capitis, including kerion); *Trichophyton, Microsporum, Epidermophyton* spp	Griseofulvin ultramicrosized 10–15 mg/kg/day or microsized 20–25 mg/kg/day once daily PO for 1–2 mo or longer (AII) (taken with milk or fatty foods to augment absorption) For kerion, treat concurrently with prednisone (1–2 mg/kg/day for 1–2 wk) (AIII)	No need to routinely follow liver function tests in normal healthy children taking griseofulvin. 2.5% selenium sulfide shampoo, or 2% ketoconazole shampoo, 2–3 times/wk should be used concurrently to prevent recurrences. Alternatives: itraconazole soln 5 mg/kg PO qd, or terbinafine PO; or fluconazole PO
– Tinea corporis (infection of trunk/limbs/face) – Tinea cruris (infection of the groin) – Tinea pedis (infection of the toes/feet)	Alphabetic order of topical agents: butenafine, ciclopirox, clotrimazole, econazole, haloprogin, ketoconazole, miconazole, naftifine, oxiconazole, sertaconazole, sulconazole, terbinafine, and tolnaftate (AII); apply daily for 4 wk	For unresponsive tinea lesions, use griseofulvin PO in dosages provided above; fluconazole PO, itraconazole PO; OR terbinafine PO. For tinea pedis: Terbinafine PO or itraconazole PO are preferred over other oral agents. Keep skin as clean and dry as possible, particularly for tinea cruris and tinea pedis.
– Tinea unguium (onychomycosis)	Topical 8% ciclopirox nail lacquer soln applied daily for 6–12 mo (AII); OR itraconazole 5 mg/kg PO soln q24h (AII)	Recurrence or partial response common. Alternative: terbinafine PO 500 mg daily (adult dosage) for 1 wk per mo for 3 mo (hands) or 6–12 mo (toes) until new nail growth
– Tinea versicolor (also pityriasis versicolor) (*Malassezia furfur*)	Apply topically: selenium sulfide 2.5% lotion or 1% shampoo daily, leave on 30 min, then rinse; for 7 d, then monthly for 6 mo (AIII); OR ciclopirox 1% cream for 4 wk (BII); OR terbinafine 1% soln (BII); OR ketoconazole 2% shampoo daily for 5 days (BII) For small lesions, topical clotrimazole, econazole, haloprogin, ketoconazole, miconazole, or naftifine	For lesions that fail to clear with topical therapy, or for extensive lesions: Fluconazole PO or itraconazole PO are equally effective. Recurrence common.

9. Preferred Therapy for Specific Viral Pathogens

NOTE

- **Abbreviations:** ACV, acyclovir; adamantanes, amantadine and rimantadine; bid, twice daily; CA, chronologic age; CDC, Centers for Disease Control and Prevention; CMV, cytomegalovirus; EBV, Epstein-Barr virus; FDA, US Food and Drug Administration; GA, gestational age; G-CSF, granulocyte-colony stimulating factor; HAART, highly active antiretroviral therapy; HIV, human immunodeficiency virus; HSV, herpes simplex virus; IG, immune globulin; IFN, interferon; NAI, neuraminadase inhibitors (oseltamivir, zanamivir, peramivir); NRTI, nucleoside analog reverse transcriptase inhibitor; qd, once daily; qid, 4 times daily; tid, 3 times daily; VZV, varicella-zoster virus.

Infection	Therapy (evidence grade)	Comments
Adenovirus (pneumonia or disseminated infection in immunocompromised hosts)	Cidofovir and ribavirin are active in vitro, but no prospective clinical data exist and cidofovir has significant toxicity; contact an infectious diseases specialist for current strategy.	The orally bioavailable lipophilic derivative of cidofovir, CMX001, is under investigation for the treatment of adenovirus in immunocompromised hosts. It is not yet commercially available.
Cytomegalovirus		
– Neonatal	See Chapter 5.	
– Immunocompromised (HIV, chemotherapy, transplant-related)	For induction: ganciclovir 10 mg/kg/day IV div q12h for 14–21 days For maintenance: 5 mg/kg IV q24h or 1 g PO tid (adults). Duration dependent on degree of immunosuppression (AII). CMV hyperimmune globulin may decrease morbidity in bone marrow transplant patients with CMV pneumonia (AII).	Use foscarnet or cidofovir for ganciclovir-resistant strains; for HIV-positive children on HAART, CMV may resolve without therapy. Also used for prevention of CMV disease post-transplant for 100–120 days. Limited data on oral valganciclovir in neonates (32 mg/kg/day PO div bid) and children dosing by body surface area (BSA) (dose [mg] = 7 × BSA × creatinine clearance)
– Prophylaxis of infection in immunocompromised hosts	Ganciclovir 5 mg/kg IV daily (or 3 times/wk) (started at engraftment for stem cell transplant patients) (BII)	Neutropenia is a complication with GCV prophylaxis and may be addressed with G-CSF. Both prophylaxis and preemptive strategies are effective; neither has been shown clearly superior to the other.
Epstein-Barr virus		
– Mononucleosis, encephalitis	Limited data suggest clinical benefit of valacyclovir in adolescents for mononucleosis (3 g/day div tid for 14 days) (CIII) For EBV encephalitis: ganciclovir IV OR acyclovir IV (AIII)	No prospective data on benefits of acyclovir IV or ganciclovir IV in EBV clinical infections of normal hosts
– Post-transplant lymphoproliferative disorder (PTLD)	Ganciclovir (AIII)	Decrease immune suppression if possible, as this has the most impact on control of EBV; rituximab, methotrexate have been used but without controlled data. Preemptive treatment with GCV may decrease PTLD in solid organ transplants.

Hepatitis B virus (chronic)	IFN-alpha 6 million IU/m² 3 times/wk for 16–24 wk for children 1–18 y; OR lamivudine 3 mg/kg/day (max 100 mg) PO q24h for 52 wk for children ≥2 y (children coinfected with HIV and hepatitis B should use the approved dose for HIV (AII); CR adefovir for children ≥12 y (10 mg PO q24h; optimum duration of therapy unknown) (BIII); OR entecavir for children ≥15 y (0.5 mg qd in patients who have not received prior nucleoside therapy; 1 mg qc in patients who are previously treated (not first choice in this setting; optimum duration of therapy unknown)(BII)	For benign childhood chronic infection, consider no treatment. Follow to confirm benign disease. IFN has many side effects: fever, flu-like syndrome, depression, neutropenia. Alternatives: Tenofovir (adult and adolescent dose [≥12 y] 300 mg qd) Telbivudine (adult dose 600 mg qd). There are not sufficient clinical data to identify the appropriate dose for use in children. Lamivudine approved for children ≥2 y, but antiviral resistance develops on therapy in 30%. Entecavir is superior to lamivudine in the treatment of chronic HBV infection and is the most potent anti-HBV agent available.
Hepatitis C virus (chronic)	IFN-alpha 3 million IU/m²/dose, 3 times per wk for 48 wk (peg-IFN products approved for adults), AND ribavirin 15 mg/kg/day in 2 divided doses PO for 48 wk (AII)	Consider postponing treatment during childhood if liver biopsy is benign. See comments above regarding IFN. Several new hepatitis C drugs are nearing FDA approval.
Herpes simplex virus		
– Third trimester prophylaxis	Acyclovir prophylaxis for pregnant women reduces HSV recurrences and viral shedding at the time of delivery, but does not fully prevent neonatal HSV (BIII).	
– Neonatal	See Chapter 5.	
– Mucocutaneous (normal host)	Acyclovir 60–80 mg/kg/day PO div tid–qid for 5–7 days; or 15 mg/kg/day IV as 1–2 h infusion civ q8h (AII) Prophylaxis for frequent recurrence (no pediatric data): 20 mg/kg/dose given bid or tid (up to 400 mg) for 6–12 mo; then reevaluate need (AII)	Foscarnet for acyclovir-resistant strains Valacyclovir and famciclovir suspensions under investigation for children Immunocompromised hosts may require 10–14 days of therapy.
– Genital	Adult doses: acyclovir 400 mg PO tid, for 7–10 days; OR valacyclovir 1 g PO bid for 10 days; OR famciclovir 250 mg PO tid for 7–10 days (FI)	All 3 drugs have been used as prophylaxis to prevent recurrence.

Infection	Therapy (evidence grade)	Comments
Herpes simplex virus (cont)		
– Encephalitis	Acyclovir 60 mg/kg/day IV as 1–2 h infusion div q8h; for 21 days for infants ≤ 4 mo. For older infants and children, 45–60 mg/kg/day IV (AIII).	Safety of high-dose acyclovir (60 mg/kg/day) not well defined beyond the neonatal period; can be used, but monitor for neurotoxicity and nephrotoxicity
– Keratoconjunctivitis	Trifluridine (ophthalmic); idoxuridine (ophthalmic); OR ganciclovir ophthalmic gel (AII)	Treat in consultation with an ophthalmologist. Topical steroids may be helpful when used together with antiviral agents.
Human herpesvirus 6 (HHV-6)		
– Immunocompromised children	No prospective comparative data; ganciclovir 10–20 mg/kg/day IV div q12h (case report (AIII)	May require high dose to control infection; safety and efficacy not defined at high doses.
Human immunodeficiency virus (HIV)		
	Current information on HIV treatment and opportunistic infections for children is posted at http://aidsinfo.nih.gov/ContentFiles/PediatricGuidelines.pd/; other information on HIV programs is available at http://www.cdc.gov/hiv/pubs/guidelines.htm. Consult with an HIV expert, if possible, for current recommendations.	
– **Therapy of HIV infection** State-of-the-art therapy is rapidly evolving with introduction of new agents and combinations; currently there are 25 individual antiretroviral agents approved for use by the FDA, 15 of which have pediatric indications; guidelines for children and adolescents are continually updated on the AIDSINFO and CDC Web site given above.	Effective therapy (HAART) consists of ≥3 agents, including 2 nucleoside reverse transcriptase inhibitors, plus a protease inhibitor or non-nucleoside reverse transcriptase inhibitor; many different combination regimens give similar treatment outcomes; choice of agents depends on the age of the child, viral load, and extent of immune depletion, in addition to judging the child's ability to adhere to the regimen.	Assess drug toxicity (based on the agents used) and virologic/immunologic response to therapy (quantitative plasma HIV and CD4 count) initially monthly and then every 3–6 mo during the plateau phase.

– First year of life	HAART with ≥3 drugs is now recommended for all infants <12 mo. regardless of clinical status or lab values (eg, zidovudine plus lamivudine plus lopinavir/ritonavir or nevirapine) (AI)	Adherence counseling and appropriate antiretroviral formulations are critical for successful implementation.
– 1–<5 y		
Asymptomatic or mild symptoms and CD4 count ≥25% of total T cells and plasma HIV RNA <100,000 copies/mL	Consider treatment (BIII).	Expert opinion has migrated toward treatment consideration even in mild clinical situations. Treatment deferral and monitoring of clinical course, CD4 count, and plasma HIV RNA on a 3- to 4-mo basis is an option.
Asymptomatic or mild symptoms and CD4 count ≥25% of total T cells and plasma HIV RNA ≥100,000 copies/mL	Begin ≥3 drug regimen (HAART) as above (BII).	Most experts now recommend treatment in settings of high viral load.
CD4 count <25% or significant symptoms or AIDS	Begin ≥3 drug regimen (HAART) as above (AI/AII).	Any of these conditions support aggressive HAART therapy.
– 1≥5 y		
Asymptomatic or mild symptoms and CD4 count >500 cells/mm³ of total T cells and plasma HIV RNA <100,000 copies/mL	Consider treatment (CIII).	Expert opinion has migrated toward treatment consideration even in mild clinical situations. Treatment deferral and monitoring of clinical course, CD4 count, and plasma HIV RNA on a 3–4 mo basis is an option.
Asymptomatic or mild symptoms and CD4 count >500 cells/mm³ of total T cells and plasma HIV RNA ≥100,000 copies/mL	Begin ≥3 drug regimen (HAART) (BII).	Most experts now recommend treatment in settings of high viral load.
CD4 count ≤500 cells/mm³ or significant symptoms or AIDS	Begin ≥3 drug regimen (HAART) (AI/BII) as above.	Any of these conditions support aggressive HAART therapy.

Infection	Therapy (evidence grade)	Comments
Human immunodeficiency virus (HIV) (cont)		
Antiretroviral-experienced child	Consult with HIV specialist.	Consider treatment history and drug resistance testing and assess adherence.
– HIV exposures, non-occupational	Therapy recommendations for exposures available on the CDC Web site given above, based on assessment of risk of HIV exposure.	Prophylaxis remains unproven; consider individually regarding risk, time from exposure, and likelihood of adherence; prophylactic regimens administered for 4 wk.
Negligible exposure risk (urine, nasal secretions, saliva, sweat, or tears—no visible blood in secretions) OR >72 hours since exposure	Prophylaxis not recommended (BIII)	
Significant exposure risk (blood, semen, vaginal, or rectal secretions from a known HIV-infected individual) AND <72 hours since exposure	Prophylaxis recommended (BIII): combivir (zidovudine/lamivudine) or Truvada (tenofovir/emtricitabine) PLUS efavirenz or Kaletra (lopinavir/ritonavir)	Preferred prophylactic regimens – Based on treatment regimens for infected individuals – 28-day regimen In the event of poor adherence or toxicity, some experts consider 2 NRTI regimens, such as combivir (zidovudine/lamivudine) or Truvada (tenofovir/emtricitabine) (BIII).
– HIV exposure, occupational	See guidelines on CDC Web site given on page 114.	

Influenza virus

Frequent changes in recommendations have occurred recently regarding influenza due to antiviral resistance that can vary from season to season; therefore, the reader should access the AAP Web site (www.aap.org) and the CDC Web site (http://www.cdc.gov/flu/professionals/antivirals/antiviral-agents-flu.htm) for the most current, accurate information.

Influenza A and B		
– Treatment	Oseltamivir Birth–<12 mo: 3 mg/kg/dose bid 1–12 y: ≤15 kg: 30 mg, bid; 16–23 kg: 45 mg, bid; 24–40 kg: 60 mg, bid; >40 kg: 75 mg, bid ≥ 13 y: 75 mg, bid, OR Zanamivir ≥7 y 10 mg by inhalation, bid for 5 days	Oseltamivir currently is drug of choice for treatment of influenza infections. Preliminary data in premature infants (median gestational age 27.5 wk, median weight 1680 g, median age 2.5 wk) suggest 1 mg/kg/dose q12h The adamantanes, amantadine and rimantadine, currently are not effective for treatment due to near-universal resistance of influenza A.
– Chemoprophylaxis	Oseltamivir 1–12 y: Same as treatment for patients 1–12 y, except dose given qd ≥ 13 y: 75 mg, qd Zanamivir ≥5 y: 10 mg by inhalation, qd for as long as 28 days (community outbreaks) or 10 days (household setting)	Oseltamivir currently is drug of choice for chemoprophylaxis of influenza infection. The adamantanes, amantadine and rimantadine, currently are not effective for chemoprophylaxis due to near-universal resistance of influenza A.
Measles	No prospective data on antiviral therapy. Ribavirin is active against measles virus in vitro. Vitamin A is beneficial to children who may be deficient (qd dosing for 2 days): for children ≥1 y: 200,000 IU; for infants 6–12 mo: 100,000 IU; for infants <6 mo: 50,000 IU. (BII)	IG prophylaxis for exposed, susceptible children: 0.25 mL/kg IM; and for immunocompromised children: 0.5 mL/kg (max 15 mL) IM

Infection	Therapy (evidence grade)	Comments
Respiratory syncytial virus (RSV)		
- Therapy (severe disease in compromised host)	Ribavirin (6-g vial to make 20 mg/mL solution in sterile water), aerosolized over 18–20 h daily for 3–5 days (BII)	Aerosol ribavirin provides a small benefit and should only be used for life-threatening infection with RSV. Airway reactivity with inhalation precludes routine use.
- Palivizumab (Synagis) prophylaxis for high-risk infants (AII) (for definition of high risk see comment)	Palivizumab (Synagis, a monoclonal antibody) 15 mg/kg IM monthly. For all high-risk groups except premature infants with GA between 32 and 35 wk, a maximum of 5 doses should be provided during the RSV season, with the first dose given on November 1, and the last dose on March 1 (currently defined as the RSV season for most of the US). For infants with GA between 32–<35 wk, a maximum of 3 doses should be provided during the RSV season. No infants should routinely receive a dose of palivizumab after the March 1 dose.	Palivizumab will not treat an active infection. In Florida, the RSV season lasts 5 months, but starts earlier than in the rest of the US. 1. Infants <24 mo with chronic lung disease who are receiving or have received medical therapy (oxygen, bronchodilator, diuretic, or corticosteroid therapy) within 6 months before start of the RSV season (since May 1) 2. Infants <24 mo with hemodynamically significant congenital heart disease (congestive heart failure requiring therapy, moderate to severe pulmonary hypertension, cyanotic heart disease) 3. Infants with congenital abnormalities of the airway or a neuromuscular disorder, who will be <12 mo on November 1 4. Extremely premature infants: GA <28 wk, and CA <12 mo on November 1 5. Very premature infants: GA 29–<32 wk (31 wk 6 days), and CA <6 mo on November 1 6. Premature infants: GA between 32 wk (32 wk 0 days) to <35 wk (34 wk 6 days), and CA <3 mo on November 1, AND 1 of 2 additional risk factors should be present to receive palivizumab: child care attendance; or a sibling <5 y.

Varicella-zoster virus		
– Infection in a normal host	Acyclovir 80 mg/kg/day (max 3.2 g/day) PO div qid for 5 days (A)	The sooner antiviral therapy can be started, the greater the impact.
– Severe primary chickenpox, disseminated infection (cutaneous, pneumonia, encephalitis, hepatitis); immunocompromised host with primary chickenpox or disseminated zoster	Acyclovir 30 mg/kg/day IV as 1–2 h infusion div q8h; for 10 days (acyclovir doses of 45–50 mg/kg/day in 3 divided doses IV should be used for disseminated or central nervous system infection). Dosing can also be provided as: 1,500 mg/m²/day IV div q8h. Duration in immunocompromised children: 7–14 days, based on clinical response (AII).	Valacyclovir, famciclovir, foscarnet also active

10. Preferred Therapy for Specific Parasitic Pathogens

NOTES

- For some parasitic diseases, therapy may be available only from the CDC, as noted. Consultation is available from the CDC for parasitic telediagnostic services (http://dpd.cdc.gov/dpdx/Default.htm), parasitic disease testing, and experimental therapy at 404/639-3670; for malaria, 770/488-7788 (or 7100). Antiparasitic drugs available from the CDC can be viewed and requested at http://www.cdc.gov/ncidod/srp/drugs/formulary.html.

- **Abbreviations:** AFB, acid-fast bacteria; bid, twice daily; BP, blood pressure; CDC, Centers for Disease Control and Prevention; CNS, central nervous system; CSF, cerebrospinal fluid; DEC, diethylcarbamazine; div, divided; ECG, electrocardiogram; FDA, US Food and Drug Administration; G6PD, glucose-6-phosphate dehydrogenase; GI, gastrointestinal; HAART, highly active antiretroviral therapy; HIV, human immunodeficiency virus; IM, intramuscular; IV, intravenous; PO, orally; qd, once daily; qid, 4 times daily; qod, every other day; tid, 3 times daily; tab, tablet; TMP/SMX, trimethroprim/sulfamethoxazole; UV, ultraviolet.

Disease/Organism	Treatment	Comments
AMEBIASIS		
ENTERITIS/LIVER ABSCESS		
Entamoeba histolytica		
– Asymptomatic carrier	Paromomycin 30 mg/kg/day PO div tid for 7 days; OR iodoquinol 30–40 mg/kg/day (max 2 g) PO div tid for 20 days; OR diloxanide furoate (not commercially available in the US) 20 mg/kg/day PO div tid for 10 days (CII)	Follow-up stool examination to ensure eradication of carriage; screen/treat positive close contacts.
– Mild to moderate colitis	Metronidazole 30–40 mg/kg/day PO div tid for 10 days; OR tinidazole 50 mg/kg/day PO (max 2 g) qd for 3 days FOLLOWED by paromomycin or iodoquinol as above to eliminate cysts (BII)	Avoid antimotility drugs, steroids. Take tinidazole with food to decrease GI side effects; if unable to take tablets, pharmacists can crush tablets and mix with syrup. Nitazoxanide (see *Giardia*) may also be effective.
– Severe colitis, liver abscess	Metronidazole 35–40 mg/kg/day IV q8h, switch to PO when tolerated, for 10 days; OR tinidazole (age ≥3 y) 50 mg/kg/day PO (max 2 g) qd for 5 days FOLLOWED by paromomycin or iodoquinol as above to eliminate cysts (BII)	Serologic assays >95% positive in extraintestinal amebiasis. Percutaneous or surgical drainage may be indicated for large liver abscesses or inadequate response to medical therapy. Chloroquine plus metronidazole or tinidazole followed by luminal agent considered alternative for liver abscess.
MENINGOENCEPHALITIS		
Naegleria, Acanthamoeba, Balamuthia, Hartmanella spp	Amphotericin B 1.5 mg/kg/day IV in 2 doses for 3 days then 1 mg/kg/day for 6 days plus 1.5 mg/day intrathecally for 2 days, then 1 mg/day qod for 8 days; consider alternative 1–1.5 mg/kg/day qd for 3–4 wk or longer, PLUS azithromycin for Naegleria	Treatment outcomes usually unsuccessful; early therapy (even before diagnostic confirmation if indicated) may improve survival. *Acanthamoeba* may be susceptible in vitro to ketoconazole, flucytosine, and pentamidine; voriconazole and miltefosine active against *Acanthamoeba* (alone or in combination with pentamidine). *Balamuthia* may be susceptible in vitro to pentamidine, azithromycin/clarithromycin, fluconazole, sulfadiazine, and flucytosine (CIII). Surgical resection of CNS lesions may be beneficial. Keratitis should be evaluated by an ophthalmologist.

Ancylostoma caninum	See EOSINOPHILIC COLITIS.	
Ancylostoma duodenale	See HOOKWORM.	
ANGIOSTRONGYLIASIS		
Angiostrongylus cantonensis	Mebendazole 100 mg PO bid for 5 days OR albendazole 20 mg/kg/day PO div bid for 9 days (CIII)	Most patients recover without antiparasitic therapy; treatment may provoke severe neurologic symptoms. Corticosteroids, analgesics, and repeat lumbar puncture may be of benefit.
Angiostrongylus costaricensis	Mebendazole 200–400 mg PO tid for 10 days; OR thiabendazole 50–75 mg/kg/day (max 3 g) PO div tid for 3 days (CII)	
ASCARIASIS (*Ascaris lumbricoides*)	Albendazole 400 mg PO once (BI) OR mebendazole 100 mg PO bid for 3 days (alternative, 500 mg once) (BII) OR ivermectin 150–200 µg/kg PO once (CII)	Follow-up stool ova and parasite exam after therapy not essential. Take albendazole with food.
BABESIOSIS (*Babesia* spp)	Clindamycin 30 mg/kg/day PO div tid, PLUS quinine 25 mg/kg/day PO div tid for 7 days (BII); OR atovaquone 40 mg/kg/day div bid, PLUS azithromycin 12 mg/kg/day for 7 days (CII)	Exchange blood transfusion may be of benefit for severe disease.
Balantidium coli	Tetracycline (patient >7 y) 40 mg/kg/day PO div qid for 10 days (max 2 g/day) (BII); OR metronidazole 35–50 mg/kg/day PO div tid for 5 days OR iodoquinol 40 mg/kg/day (max 2 g/day) PO div tid for 20 days (CI)	Repeated stool examination may be needed for diagnosis; prompt stool examination may increase detection of rapidly degenerating trophozoites.
Baylisascaris procyonis (raccoon roundworm)	For CNS infection, albendazole 25–40 mg/kg/day PO div q12h AND high-dose corticosteroid therapy (CIII)	Therapy generally unsuccessful to prevent fatal outcome or severe neurologic sequelae once CNS disease present. Steroids may be of value in decreasing inflammation with therapy of CNS or ocular infection. Retinal worms may be killed by direct photocoagulation. Consider prophylactic albendazole for children who may have ingested soil contaminated with raccoon feces.

Disease/Organism	Treatment	Comments
Blastocystis hominis	Metronidazole 30 mg/kg/day PO div tid for 10 days; OR iodoquinol 40 mg/kg/day (max 2 g) PO div tid for 20 days; OR nitazoxanide (as for Cryptosporidium) (CII)	Normal hosts may not need therapy; reexamination of stool for other parasites (eg, Giardia) may be of value. Metronidazole resistance may occur.
CHAGAS DISEASE (Trypanosoma cruzi)	See TRYPANOSOMIASIS.	
Clonorchis sinensis	See FLUKES.	
CRYPTOSPORIDIOSIS (Cryptosporidium parvum)	Nitazoxanide, age 12–47 mo, 5 mL (100 mg) bid for 3 days; age 4–11 y, 10 mL (200 mg) bid for 3 days (BII); OR paromomycin 30 mg/kg/day div bid-qid (CII); OR azithromycin 10 mg/kg/day for 5 days (CII); repeated treatment courses may be needed	Disease may be self-limited in normal hosts. In HIV-infected patients not receiving HAART, medical therapy may have limited efficacy.
CUTANEOUS LARVA MIGRANS or **CREEPING ERUPTION** (dog and cat hookworm) Ancylostoma caninum, Ancylostoma braziliense, Uncinaria stenocephala	Albendazole 15 mg/kg PO qd for 3 days (BII); OR ivermectin 200 µg/kg PO once (BII)	
Cyclospora spp (cyanobacterium-like agent)	TMP/SMX (10 mg TMP/kg/day) PO div bid for 5–10 days (BIII); OR ciprofloxacin 30 mg/kg/day div bid for 7days	HIV-infected patients may require higher doses/longer therapy.
CYSTICERCOSIS (Cysticercus cellulosae)	Albendazole 15 mg/kg/day PO div bid (max 800 mg/day) for 8–30 days (CII); OR praziquantel 50–100 mg/kg/day PO div tid for 15–30 days (phenytoin decreases praziquantel conc) (CII)	For CNS disease with multiple lesions, give steroids and anticonvulsants before first dose; for CNS disease with few lesions, steroid pretreatment not required. Contraindicated for eye or spinal cord lesions (surgery as indicated). Treatment controversial, especially for single lesion disease.
DIENTAMEBIASIS (Dientamoeba fragilis)	Paromomycin 25 mg/kg/day PO div tid for 7 days; OR iodoquinol 40 mg/kg/day (max 2 g) PO div tid for 20 days; OR metronidazole 30 mg/kg/day PO div tid for 10 days (BII)	Asymptomatic colonization more common in adults than children.

Diphyllobothrium latum	See TAPEWORMS.
ECHINOCOCCOSIS	
Echinococcus granulosus, Echinococcus multilocularis	Albendazole 15 mg/kg/day PO div bid (max 800 mg/day) for 1–6 mo alone (CIII), or combined with praziquantel 50–75 mg/kg/day daily (BIII) for 5–14 d ± once weekly dose for additional 3–6 mo	Surgical excision may be the only reliable therapy; ultrasound-guided percutaneous aspiration-injection-reaspiration (PAIR) plus albendazole may be effective for hepatic hydatid cysts.
Entamoeba histolytica	See AMEBIASIS.
Enterobius vermicularis	See PINWORMS.
Fasciola hepatica	See FLUKES.
EOSINOPHILIC COLITIS (Ancylostoma caninum)	Mebendazole 100 mg PO bid for 3 days; OR albendazole 15 mg/kg/day PO div bid (max 400 mg/day) (BIII)	Endoscopic removal may be considered if medical treatment not successful.
EOSINOPHILIC MENINGITIS	See ANGIOSTRONGYLIASIS.
FILARIASIS		Ivermectin may be effective for killing *Wuchereria, Brugia,* and *Loa loa* microfilariae; in heavy infections or when coinfection with *O volvulus* possible, consider ivermectin initially to reduce microfilaremia before giving DEC (decreased risk of encephalopathy or severe allergic or febrile reaction).
– River blindness (Onchocerca volvulus)	Ivermectin 150 μg/kg PO once (AIII); repeat q6–12 mo until asymptomatic and no chronic, ongoing exposure	Antihistamines or corticosteroids are of major benefit for allergic reactions.
– Wuchereria bancrofti, Brugia malayi, Mansonella streptocerca	*W bancrofti, B malayi, M streptocerca:* DEC (from CDC) 1 mg/kg PO after food on day 1: then 3 mg/kg/day div tid on day 2; then 3–6 mg/kg/day div tid on day 3; then 6 mg/kg/day div tid on days 4–14 (AII)	
Mansonella ozzardi	Ivermectin 150 μg/kg PO once may be effective	DEC not reported to be effective
Mansonella perstans	Albendazole 400 mg PO bid for 10 days; mebendazole 100 mg PO bid for 30 days	

Disease/Organism	Treatment	Comments
Loa loa	DEC (from CDC) as above, then 9 mg/kg/day div tid on days 14–21 (AII)	
Tropical pulmonary eosinophilia (TPE)	DEC (from CDC) 6 mg/kg/day PO tid for 14 days; antihistamines/corticosteroids for allergic reactions (CII)	
FLUKES		
Chinese liver fluke (*Clonorchis sinensis*) and others (*Fasciolopsis, Heterophyes, Metagonimus, Metorchis, Nanophyetus, Opisthorchis*)	Praziquantel 75 mg/kg PO tid for 2 days (BII); OR albendazole 10 mg/kg/day PO qd for 7 days (CIII)	Take praziquantel with liquids and food.
Lung fluke (*Paragonimus westermani* and other *Paragonimus* lung flukes)	Praziquantel 75 mg/kg PO div tid for 2 days (BII)	Triclabendazole (5 mg/kg qd for 3 days or 10 mg/kg bid for 1 day) may also be effective; triclabendazole should be taken with food to facilitate absorption.
Sheep liver fluke (*Fasciola hepatica*)	Triclabendazole (from CDC) 10 mg/kg PO once (BII) OR bithionol (from CDC) 30–50 mg/kg PO div qid on alternate days for 10–15 doses (BII); OR nitazoxanide PO (take with food), age 12–47 mo 100 mg/dose bid for 7 days; age 4–11 y, 200 mg/dose bid for 7 days; age ≥12 y, 1 tab (500 mg)/dose bid for 7 days (CII)	
GIARDIASIS (*Giardia lamblia*)	Metronidazole 30–40 mg/kg/day PO div tid for 7–10 days (BII); OR nitazoxanide PO (take with food), age 12–47 mo 100 mg/dose bid for 7 days; age 4–11 y, 200 mg/dose bid for 7 days; age ≥12 y, 1 tab (500 mg)/dose bid for 7 days (BII); OR tinidazole 50 mg/kg/day (max 2 g) for 1 day (BII)	If therapy inadequate, another course of the same agent usually curative. Alternatives: furazolidone 6 mg/kg/day in 4 doses for 7–10 days; OR paromomycin 30 mg/kg/day div tid for 5–10 days; OR albendazole 10 mg/kg/day PO for 5 days (CII) Prolonged courses may be needed for immunocompromising conditions (eg, hypogammaglobulinemia). Treatment of asymptomatic carriers not usually recommended.

HOOKWORM		
Necator americanus, Ancylostoma duodenale	Albendazole 10 mg/kg (max 400 mg) once (repeat dose may be necessary) (BII); OR mebendazole 100 mg PO bid for 3 day (alternative, 500 mg once (BII); OR pyrantel pamoate 11 mg/kg (max 1 g/day) (BII) PO qd for 3 days	Perform repeat stool examination 2 weeks after treatment, re-treat If positive.
Hymenolepis nana	See TAPEWORMS.	
ISOSPORIASIS *(Isospora belli;* now also known as *Cystoisosporiasis*	TMP/SMX (10 mg TMP/kg/day PO div qid for 10 days; then 5 mg TMP/kg/day PO div bid for 3 wk; pyrimethamine may be effective (CII) HIV-infected children may need longer courses of therapy (consider long-term maintenance therapy for multiple relapses).	Infection often self-limited in immunocompetent hosts. Repeated stool examinations and special techniques (eg, modified AFB staining or UV microscopy) may be needed to detect low oocyst numbers.
LEISHMANIASIS, including kala azar		
Leishmania spp	Visceral: liposomal amphotericin E, 3 mg/kg/day on days 1–5, day 14, and day 21 (BII); OR sodium stibogluconate (from CDC) 20 mg/kg/day IM, IV for 20–28 days (or longer) (BII); OR miltefosine 2.5 mg/kg/day PO (max 150 mg/day) for 28 days (BII); OR amphotericin E 1 mg/kg/day IV daily for 15–20 days or every second day for 4–3 wk (BIII); OR paromomycin sulfate 15 mg/kg/day IM for 21 days (BII) Cutaneous: sodium stibogluconate 20 mg/kg/day IM, IV for 20 days (BIII); OR miltefosine (as above) (BII); OR pentamidine isethionate 2–4 mg/kg/day IM daily or every second day for 4 days (BII) Mucosal: sodium stibogluconate 20 mg/kg/day IM, IV for 28 days; OR amphotericin B 0.5–1 mg/kg/day IV daily for 15–20 days or every second day for 4–8 wk; OR miltefosine (as above)	Consult with tropical medicine specialist if unfamiliar with leishmaniasis. Patients infected in south Asia (especially India, Nepal) should receive non-antimonial regimens because of high rates of resistance. Azoles (eg, fluconazole, ketoconazole) may be effective for cutaneous disease but should be avoided in treating mucosal or visceral disease. Topical paromomycin (15%) applied twice daily for 10–20 days may be considered for cutaneous leishmaniasis in areas where the potential for mucosal disease is rare.

Disease/Organism	Treatment	Comments
LICE		
Pediculus capitis or humanus, Phthirus pubis	Follow manufacturer's instructions for topical use: permethrin 1% (BII); OR malathion 0.5% (BIII); OR pyrethrins; OR lindane; for topical therapies repeat in 1 wk; OR ivermectin 200 µg/kg PO once	Launder bedding and clothing; for eyelash infestation, use petrolatum; for head lice, remove nits with comb designed for that purpose. Administration of 3 doses of ivermectin (1 dose/wk separately by weekly intervals) may be needed to eradicate infection.
MALARIA		
Plasmodium falciparum, Plasmodium vivax, Plasmodium ovale, Plasmodium malariae	CDC Physician's Malaria Hotline 770/488-7788 (or 7100); online information at http://www.cdc.gov/malaria/. Consult tropical medicine specialist if unfamiliar with malaria.	No antimalarial drug provides absolute protection against malaria; fever after return from an endemic area should prompt an immediate evaluation. Emphasize personal protective measures (insecticides, bed nets, clothing, avoidance of dusk-dawn mosquito exposures).
Prophylaxis		
For areas with chloroquine-resistant *P falciparum* or *P vivax*	Atovaquone-proguanil (A-P): 11–20 kg, 1 pediatric tab (62.5 mg atovaquone/25 mg proguanil); 21–30 kg, 2 pediatric tabs; 31–40 kg, 3 pediatric tabs; >40 kg, 1 adult tab (250 mg atovaquone/100 mg proguanil) PO daily starting 1–2 days before travel and continuing 7 days after last exposure; for children <10 kg, data on A-P are limited (BII); OR mefloquine: for children <5 kg, 5 mg/kg; 5–9 kg, 1/8 tab; 10–19 kg, 1/4 tab; 20–30 kg, 1/2 tab; 31–45 kg, 3/4 tab; >45 kg (adult dose) 1 tab PO once weekly starting 1 wk before arrival in area and continuing for 4 wk after leaving area (BII); OR doxycycline (patients >7 y): 2 mg/kg (max 100 mg) PO daily starting 1–2 days before arrival in area and continuing for 4 wk after leaving area (BII); OR primaquine (check for G6PD deficiency before administering): 0.5 mg/kg base daily starting 1–2 days before travel and continuing for 2 days after last exposure (BII)	Avoid mefloquine for persons with a history of seizures or psychosis, active depression, or cardiac conduction abnormalities. *P falciparum* resistance to mefloquine exists along the borders between Thailand and Myanmar and Thailand and Cambodia, Myanmar and China, and Myanmar and Laos; isolated resistance has been reported in southern Vietnam. Take doxycycline with adequate fluids to avoid esophageal irritation and food to avoid GI side effects; use sunscreen and avoid excessive sun exposure.

For areas without chloroquine-resistant *P falciparum* or *P vivax*	Chloroquine phosphate 5 mg base/kg (max 300 mg base) PO once weekly, beginning 1 wk before arrival in area and continuing for 4 wk after leaving area (available in suspension outside the US and Canada) (AII) For heavy or prolonged (months) exposure to mosquitoes: treat with primaquine (check for G6PD deficiency before administering) 0.3–0.6 mg base/kg PO qd with final 2 wk of chloroquine for prevention of relapse with *P ovale* or *P vivax*

Disease/Organism	Treatment	Comments
Treatment of disease		
– Chloroquine-resistant *P falciparum* or *P vivax*	*Oral therapy:* atovaquone-proguanil: for children <5 kg, data limited; 5–8 kg, 2 pediatric tabs (62.5 mg atovaquone/25 mg proguanil) PO qd for 3 days; 9–10 kg, 3 pediatric tabs qd for 3 days; 11–20 kg, 1 adult tab (250 mg atovaquone/ 100 mg proguanil) qd for 3 days; 21–30 kg, 2 adult tabs qd for 3 days; 31–40 kg, 3 adult tabs qd for 3 days; >40 kg, 4 adult tabs qd for 3 days OR quinine 25 mg/kg/day (max 2 g/day) PO div tid for 3–7 days AND doxycycline (patients >7 y) 2 mg/kg/day for 7 days, or pyrimethamine-sulfadoxine: <1 y, 1/4 tab; 1–3 y, 1/2 tab; 4–8 y, 1 tab; 9–14 y, 2 tab; >14 y, 3 tabs as a single dose on last day of quinine; or clindamycin 30 mg/kg/day div tid (max 900 mg tid) for 5 days; OR artemether/lumefantrine 6 doses over 3 days at 0, 8, 24, 36, 48, and 60 h; <15 kg, 1 tab/dose; 15–25 kg, 2 tabs/dose; 25–35 kg, 3 tabs/dose; >35 kg, 4 tabs/dose (not available in US) (BII) *Parenteral therapy* (check with CDC): quinidine 10 mg/kg (max 600 mg) IV (1 h infusion in normal saline) followed by continuous infusion of 0.02 mg/kg/min until oral therapy can be given (after 48-h therapy, decrease dose by 1/3 to 1/2); (BII) alternative: artesunate 2.4 mg/kg/dose IV for 3 days at 0, 12, 24, 48, and 72 h (from CDC) (B1) For prevention of relapse with *P vivax, P ovale:* primaquine (check for G6PD deficiency before administering) 0.3–0.6 mg base/kg/day PO for 14 days	Consider exchange blood transfusion for >10% parasitemia, altered mental status, pulmonary edema, or renal failure. Mild disease may be treated with oral antimalarial drugs; severe disease (impaired level of consciousness, convulsion, hypotension, or parasitemia >5%) should be treated parenterally. Avoid mefloquine for treatment of malaria if possible given higher dose and increased incidence of adverse events. Do not use primaquine during pregnancy; for relapses of primaquine-resistant *P vivax* or *P ovale,* consider retreating with primaquine 30 mg (base) for 28 days. Continuously monitor ECG, BP, and glucose in patients receiving quinidine. Use artesunate for when quinidine intolerance, treatment failure, or lack of availability; http://www.cdc.gov/malaria/ resources/pdf/treatmenttable.pdf; artemisinins should be used in combination with other drugs to avoid resistance.

– Chloroquine-susceptible P falciparum, chloroquine-susceptible P vivax, P ovale, P malariae	Oral therapy: chloroquine 10 mg/kg base (max 600 mg base) PO then 5 mg/kg 6 h, 24 h, and 48 h after initial dose Parenteral therapy: quinidine, as above See above for prevention of relapse due to P vivax and P ovale.	
Paragonimus westermani	See FLUKES.	
PINWORMS (Enterobius vermicularis)	Mebendazole 100 mg PO once (BII); OR albendazole 10 mg/kg (max 400 mg) PO once (BII); OR pyrantel pamoate 11 mg/kg (max 1 g) PO once (BII); repeat treatment in 2 wk	Treatment of entire household (and if this fails, consider close child care/school contacts) often recommended; re-treatment of contacts after 2 wk may be needed to prevent reinfection.
PNEUMOCYSTIS	See Chapter 8, Specific Fungal Pathogens, Pneumocystis.	
SCABIES (Sarcoptes scabei)	Permethrin 5% cream applied to entire body (including scalp in infants), left on for 8–14 h then bathe (BII); OR lindane lotion applied to body below neck, leave on overnight bathe in am (BII); OR ivermectin 200 µg/kg PO once (BII)	Launder bedding and clothing. Reserve lindane for patients who do not respond to other therapy. Treatment may need to be repeated in 10–14 days.
SCHISTOSOMIASIS (Schistosoma haematobium, Schistosoma japonicum, Schistosoma mansoni, Schistosoma mekongi, Schistosoma intercalatum)	Praziquantel 40 (for S haematobium and S mansoni) or 60 (for S japonicum and S mekongi) mg/kg/day PO div bid (if 40 mg/day) tid (if 60 mg/day) for 1 day (AI); OR oxamniquine (not commercially available in the US) 15 mg/kg PO once (West Africa, Brazil), or 40–60 mg/kg/day for 2–3 days (most of Africa) for praziquantel-resistant S mansoni infections (BI)	Take praziquantel with food and liquids.
STRONGYLOIDIASIS (Strongyloides stercoralis)	Ivermectin 200 µg/kg PO qd for 1–2 days (BII); OR thiabendazole 50 mg/kg/day (max 3 g/day) PO div bid for 2 days (5 days or longer for disseminated disease) (BII)	Albendazole is less effective but may be adequate if longer courses used.

Disease/Organism	Treatment	Comments
TAPEWORMS		
– *Cysticercus cellulosae*	See CYSTICERCOSIS.	
– *Echinococcus granulosus*	See ECHINOCOCCOSIS.	
– *Taenia saginata, T solium, Hymenolepis nana, Diphyllobothrium latum, Dipylidium caninum*	Praziquantel 5–10 mg/kg PO once (25 mg/kg once for *H nana*) (BIII); OR niclosamide tab 50 mg/kg PO once, chewed thoroughly (all but *H nana*)	
TOXOPLASMOSIS (*Toxoplasma gondii*)	Pyrimethamine 2 mg/kg/day PO div bid for 3 days (max 100 mg) then 1 mg/kg/day (max 25 mg) PO qd AND sulfadiazine 120 mg/kg/day PO div qid (max 6 g/day); with supplemental folinic acid and leucovorin 10–25 mg with each dose of pyrimethamine (AI) See Chapter 5 for congenital infection. For treatment in pregnancy, spiramycin 50–100 mg/kg/day PO div qid (available as investigational therapy through the FDA at 301/827-2335) (CII)	Treatment continued for 2 wk after resolution of illness; concurrent corticosteroids given for ocular or CNS infection. Prolonged therapy if HIV positive. Take pyrimethamine with food to decrease GI adverse effects; sulfadiazine should be taken on an empty stomach with adequate liquids. Atovaquone plus pyrimethamine may be effective for patients intolerant of sulfa-containing drugs.
TRAVELER'S DIARRHEA	Azithromycin 10 mg/kg qd for 3–5 days (BIII); OR rifaximin 200 mg PO tid for 3 days (ages ≥12 y) (BIII); OR ciprofloxacin (BII); OR cefixime (CII)	Azithromycin preferable to ciprofloxacin for travelers to SE Asia given high prevalence of quinolone-resistant *Campylobacter*. Rifaximin may not be as efficacious for *Shigella* and other enterics in patients with bloody diarrhea and invasive infection.
TRICHINELLOSIS (*Trichinella spiralis*)	Mebendazole 200–400 mg PO tid for 3 days, then 400–500 mg tid for 10 days (BIII); OR albendazole 20 mg/kg/day (max 400 mg/dose) PO div bid for 8–14 days (BII)	Neither drug effective for larvae already in muscles. Anti-inflammatory drugs, steroids for CNS or cardiac involvement or severe symptoms.
TRICHOMONIASIS (*Trichomonas vaginalis*)	Metronidazole 40 mg/kg (max 2 g) PO for 1 dose, or metronidazole 500 mg PO bid for 7 days (AII); OR tinidazole 50 mg/kg (max 2 g) PO for 1 dose (BII)	Treat sex partners simultaneously. Metronidazole resistance occurs and may be treated with higher-dose metronidazole or tinidazole.

Trichuris trichiura	See WHIPWORM.	
TRYPANOSOMIASIS		
– Chagas Disease (*Trypanosoma cruzi*)	Nifurtimox PO (from CDC): children 1–10 y, 15–20 mg/kg/day div qid for 90–120 days; 11–16 y, 12.5–15 mg/kg/day div qid for 90–120 days; 17 y and older: 8–10 mg/kg/day div tid–qid for 90–120 days (BIII); OR benznidazole PO (not commercially available in the US): children <12 y 10 mg/kg/day div bid for 30–90 days; 12 y and older: 5–7 mg/kg/day div bid for 30–60 days (BIII)	Therapy recommended for acute and congenital infection, reactivated infection, and chronic infection in children aged <18 y. Take benznidazole with meals to avoid GI adverse effects. Interferon-γ in addition to nifurtimox may shorten acute disease duration.
– Sleeping Sickness *Trypanosoma brucei gambiense* (West African) *T brucei rhodesiense* (East African) Acute (hemolymphatic) stage	*Tb gambiense*: pentamidine isethionate 4 mg/kg/day (max 300 mg) IM for 7 days (BII); *Tb rhodesiense*: suramin (from CDC) 20 mg/kg (max 1.5 g) IV on days 1, 3, 7, 14, and 21 (BIII)	Consult with tropical medicine specialist if unfamiliar with trypanosomiasis. Examination of the buffy coat of peripheral blood may be helpful. *Tb gambiense* may be found in lymph node aspirates.
Late (CNS) stage	*Tb gambiense*: eflornithine (not available commercially in the US) 400 mg/kg/day IV div q6h for 14 days (BIII); OR melarsoprol (from CDC) 2.2 mg/day (max 180 mg) IV for 10 days (BIII); *Tb rhodesiense*: melarsoprol, 2–3.6 mg/kg/day IV for 3 days; after 7 days, 3.6 mg/kg/day IV for 3 days; repeat again after 7 days; (max 180 mg); corticosteroids given with melarsopro to decrease risk of CNS toxicity	CSF examination needed for management (double-centrifuge technique recommended); perform repeat CSF examinations every 6 mo for 2 y to detect relapse.
VISCERAL LARVA MIGRANS (TOXOCARIASIS)		
Toxocara canis; *Toxocara cati*	Albendazole 15 mg/kg/day PO bid for 3–5 days (BIII). OR DEC (from CDC) 6 mg/kg/day PO div tid for 7–10 days; OR mebendazole 100–200 mg PO bid for 5 days	Some experts advocate longer therapy (eg, 20 days). Corticosteroids if severe or ocular involvement.

Disease/Organism	Treatment	Comments
WHIPWORM (TRICHURIASIS)		
Trichuris trichiura	Mebendazole 100 mg PO bid for 3 days or 500 mg once (BII); OR albendazole 400 mg PO for 3 days; OR ivermectin 200 µg/kg/day PO daily for 3 days (BII)	Stool reexamination after treatment usually not necessary.
Wuchereria bancrofti	See FILARIASIS.	

11. Alphabetic Listing of Antimicrobials

NOTES

- Higher dosages in a dose range are generally indicated for more serious illnesses.

- For most antimicrobials, a maximum dosage is provided, based on FDA reviewed and approved clinical data. However, data may be published on higher dosages than originally approved by the FDA, particularly for generic drugs (eg, the oral dosages used to treat bone and joint infections), and whenever possible, these dosages are also provided.

- For additional information on dosing in obesity, see Chapter 12. No single accurate adjustment for dosing can be made for all drug classes and tissue sites, and most published data result from single patient reports, or a study of a small group. As a rough guide, to achieve serum concentrations that are achieved in patients of normal body weight

Aminoglycosides	Start with standard mg/kg dose based on ideal body weight, then use a 40% correction factor for additional kg of weight above IBW
Vancomycin	Mg/kg dose based on total body weight, but may need to dose more frequently, as clearance is increased in obesity
Beta lactams	Mg/kg dose based on total body weight, as drugs generally distribute in all tissues and clearance is increased (variability noted among beta-lactams)
Fluoroquinolones	As with aminoglycosides, increase dose based on a 40%–45% correction factor for additional kg of weight above standard mg/kg dosing for IBW
Linezolid	Use no more than the adult maximum dose (600 mg), although some studies showed a decrease in drug exposure in obese subjects

In some situations, the benefits for treatment of a particular infection with a particular drug are greater than the potential for unknown risks at that higher dosage.

- Drugs with FDA-approved pediatric dosage, or dosages based on multiple randomized clinical trials, are given a Level of Evidence I. Dosages for which data are collected from adults, from noncomparative trials, or from small comparative trials, the Level of Evidence is II. For dosages that are based on expert or consensus opinion, or case reports, the Level of Evidence given is III.

- All commercially available dosage forms for children and adults are listed. If no oral liquid form is available, round the child's dose to the nearest value using a combination of commercially available solid dosage form strengths OR consult pharmacist for recommendations on mixing with food (eg, crushing tablets, emptying capsule contents) or the availability of a valid extemporaneously compounded liquid formulation if the child is unable to take solid dosage forms.

- **Abbreviations:** AOM, acute otitis media; bid, twice daily; BSA, body surface area; CA-MRSA, community-associated methicillin-resistant *Staphylococcus aureus;* cap, caplet; CNS, central nervous system; CMV, cytomegalovirus; CrCl, creatinine clearance; EC, enteric coated; ER, extended release; FDA, US Food and Drug Administration; hs, at bedtime; HSV, herpes simplex virus; IBW, ideal body weight; IM, intramuscular; IV, intravenous; ivpb, intravenous piggyback (premixed bag); MAC, *Mycobacterium avium* complex; oint, ointment; ophth, ophthalmic; PCP, *Pneumocystis* pneumonia; PIP, piperacillin; PK, pharmacokinetic; PO, oral; pwd, powder; soln, solution; qd, once daily; qhs, every bedtime; qid, 4 times daily; SPAG-2, small particle aerosol generator model-2; SQ, subcutaneous; susp, suspension; tab, tablet; TB, tuberculosis; TBW, total body weight; tid, 3 times daily; SMX, sulfamethoxazole; TMP, trimethoprim; top, topical; UTI, urinary tract infection; vag, vaginal; VZV, varicella-zoster virus.

A. SYSTEMIC ANTIMICROBIALS WITH DOSAGE FORMS AND USUAL DOSAGES

Generic and Trade Names	Dosage Form	Route	Dose (evidence grade)	Interval
Abacavir, Ziagen Not approved for use in infants aged <3 mo	100-mg/5-mL soln 300-mg tab	PO	16 mg/kg/day (adults 600 mg/day) (I)	q12–24h
Epzicom	Combination tab with 600 mg abacavir + 300 mg lamivudine	PO	Adolescents ≥16 y/Adults 1 tab	q24h
Trizivir	Combination tab with 300 mg abacavir, 300 mg zidovudine, 150 mg lamivudine	PO	Adolescents ≥40 kg/Adults 1 tab	q12h
Acyclovir*, Zovirax	500-, 1,000-mg vial	IV	15–60 mg/kg/day (adolescents/adults 15–30 mg/kg/day based on IBW) (I)	q8h
	200-mg/5-mL susp 200-mg cap; 400-, 800-mg tab	PO	60–80 mg/kg/day (adults 1–4 g/day) (I)	q6–8h
Albendazole, Albenza	200-mg tab	PO	15 mg/kg/day (max 800 mg/day) (I)	q12h
Amantadine*, Symmetrel	100-mg cap, tab 100-mg cap, tab 50-mg/5-mL soln	PO	5–9 mg/kg/day (max 150 mg/day if <9 y) 200 mg/day if ≥9 y (I)	q12h
Amikacin*, Amikin	500-, 1,000-mg vials, 500-mg ivpb	IV, IM	15–22.5 mg/kg/day (see Chapter 1 regarding q24h dosing) (I)	q8–24h
Amoxicillin*, Amoxil	125-, 200-, 250-, 400-mg/5-mL susp	PO	40–100 mg/kg/day if <40kg (II)	q8–12h
	125-, 200-, 250-, 400-mg chew tab	PO	Max 150 mg/kg/day divided tid for penicillin-resistant S pneumoniae otitis media (III)	q8–12h
	250-, 500-mg cap 500-, 875-mg tab	PO	>40 kg and adults 750–1,750 mg/day (I)	q8–12h
Amoxicillin extended release*, Moxatag	775-mg tab	PO	≥12 y and adults 775 mg/day	q24h

A. SYSTEMIC ANTIMICROBIALS WITH DOSAGE FORMS AND USUAL DOSAGES (cont)

Generic and Trade Names	Dosage Form	Route	Dose (evidence grade)	Interval
Amoxicillin/clavulanate*, Augmentin	**16:1** Formulation (Augmentin XR): 1,000/62.5-mg tab	PO	Adult strength	
	14:1 Formulation (Augmentin ES-600): 600/42.9-mg/5-mL susp	PO	**14:1** Formulation: 90-mg amoxicillin component/kg/day if <40 kg (I)	q12h
	7:1 Formulation: **875**/125-mg tab **200**/28.5-, **400**/57-mg chew tab; **200**/28.5-, **400**/57-mg/5-mL susp	PO	**7:1** Formulation: 25–45-mg amoxicillin component/kg/day (adults 1,750 mg/day) (I)	q12h
	4:1 Formulation: **500**/125-mg tab **125**/31.25-, **250**/62.5-mg chew tab; **125**/31.25-, **250**/62.5-mg/5-mL susp	PO	**4:1** Formulation: 20–40-mg amoxicillin component/kg/day (adults 1,500 mg/day) (I)	q8h
Amphotericin B deoxycholate (AmB-D)*, Fungizone	50-mg vial	IV	0.7–1 mg/kg (II) Adults 1–1.5 mg/kg (I)	q24h
Amphotericin B cholesteryl sulfate, Amphotec	50-, 100-mg vial	IV	3–4 mg/kg pediatric and adult dose (I)	q24h
Amphotericin B, lipid complex (AmB-LC), Abelcet	100-mg/20-mL vial	IV	5 mg/kg pediatric and adult dose (I); may push to 10 mg/kg but no data to support improved efficacy (III)	q24h
Amphotericin B, liposomal (AmB-LP), AmBisome	50-mg vial	IV	3–5 mg/kg pediatric and adult dose (I); may push to 10 mg/kg but no data to support improved efficacy (III)	q24h

Ampicillin/ampicillin trihydrate*	250-, 500-mg cap 125-, 250-mg/5-mL susp	PO	50–100 mg/kg/day if <20 kg (I) ≥20 kg and adults 1–2 g/day (I)	q6h
Ampicillin sodium*	0.125-, 0.25-, 0.5-, 1-, 2-, 10-g vial	IV, IM	50–200 mg/kg/day (I)	q6h
			300–400 mg/kg/day endocarditis/meningitis (III) Adults 2–12 g/day (I)	q4–6h
Ampicillin and sulbactam*, Unasyn	1/0.5-, 2/1-, 10/5-g vial	IV/IM	200 mg/kg/day (amp) if <40 kg (I) ≥40 kg and adults 4–8 g ampicillin/day (I)	q6h
Anidulafungin, Eraxis	50-, 100-mg vial	IV	1.5–3 mg/kg loading dose followed by 0.75–1.5 mg/kg (II) Adult loading dose 100–200 mg followed by 50–100 mg (I)	q24h
Atazanavir, Reyataz	100-, 150-, 200- 300-mg cap	PO	≥ 6 y of age: (I) If 15–<25 kg: 150 mg + ritonavir 80 mg If 25–<32 kg: 200 mg + ritonavir 100 mg If 32–<39 kg: 250 mg + ritonavir 100 mg If ≥39 kg: 300 mg + ritonavir 100 mg	q24h
Atovaquone, Mepron	750-mg/5-mL susp	PO	30 mg/kg/day if 1 to 3 mo or >24 mo (I) 45 mg/kg/day if 4–24 mo (I) Adolescents/adults 1,500 mg/day (I)	Daily dose divided q12h for PCP treatment, but given q24h for prophylaxis
Atovaquone and proguanil, Malarone	62.5/25-mg pediatric tab 250/100-mg adult tab	PO	Prophylaxis for malaria: 11–20 kg 1 ped tab, 21–30 kg 2 ped tabs, 31–40 kg 3 ped tabs, >40 kg 1 adult tab (I) Treatment: 5–8 kg 2 ped tabs, 9–10 kg 3 ped tabs, 11–20 kg 1 adult tab, 21–30 kg 2 adult tabs, 31–40 kg 3 adult tabs, >40 kg 4 adult tabs (I)	q24h

A. SYSTEMIC ANTIMICROBIALS WITH DOSAGE FORMS AND USUAL DOSAGES (cont)

Generic and Trade Names	Dosage Form	Route	Dose (evidence grade)	Interval
Azithromycin*, Zithromax, Zmax	250-, 500-, 600-mg tab 100-, 200-mg/5-mL susp 27-mg/mL extended release susp (Zmax)	PO	Otitis: 10 mg/kg/day for 1 day, then 5 mg/kg for 4 days; or 10 mg/kg/day for 3 days; or 30 mg/kg once (I) Pharyngitis: 12 mg/kg/day for 5 days (I) Sinusitis: 10 mg/kg/day for 3 days (I) Community-associated pneumonia: 10 mg/kg for 1day, then 5 mg/kg/day for 4 days or 60 mg/kg once of extended release (Zmax) susp (I) Adult single or total course dose: 1.5–2 g (I) MAC/PCP prophylaxis: 5 mg/kg/day (I) See Chapter 6 for other specific disease dosing recommendations.	q24h
Azithromycin*, Zithromax	500-mg vial	IV	10 mg/kg (II)	q24h
Aztreonam*, Azactam	1-, 2-g vial*, 1-, 2-g ivpb	IV, IM	90–120 mg/kg/day (adults 3–6 g/day) (I)	q6–8h
Aztreonam, inhalation, Cayston	75-mg soln	Inhaled	≥7 y: 75 mg/dose via Altera nebulizer (I)	q8h
Capreomycin, Capastat	1-g vial	IV, IM	15–30 mg/kg (III) Adults 1 g, max 20 mg/kg (I)	q24h
Caspofungin, Cancidas	50-, 70-mg vial	IV	70 mg/m² once, then 50 mg/m² maximum dose 70 mg (I)	q24h
Cefaclor*, Ceclor	125-, 187-, 250-, 375-mg/5-mL susp 250-, 500-mg cap, 375-, 500-mg ER tab	PO	20–40 mg/kg/day, max 1 g/day (I)	q12h
Cefadroxil*, Duricef	250-, 500-mg/5-mL susp 500-mg cap, 1-g tab	PO	30 mg/kg/day (adults 1–2 g/day) (I)	q12–24h

Cefazolin*, Ancef	0.5-, 1-, 10-, 20-g vial, 1-, 2-g vpb	IV, IM	25–100 mg/kg/day (adults 3–6 g/day) (I) For serious infections, up to 150 mg/kg/day (III)	q6-8h
Cefdinir*, Omnicef	125-, 250-mg/5-mL susp, 300-mg cap	PO	14 mg/kg/day, max 600 mg/day (I)	q24h
Cefditoren*, Spectracef	200-, 400-mg tab	PO	≥12 y and adults, 400–800 mg/day (I)	q12h
Cefepime*, Maxipime	1-, 2-g vial 1-g/50-mL 2-g/100-mL ivpb	IV, IM	100 mg/kg/day (adults 2–4 g/day) (I)	q12h
			150 mg/kg/day empiric therapy of fever with neutropenia (adults 6 g/day) (I)	q8h
Cefixime*, Suprax	100-, 200-mg/5-mL susp 400-mg tab	PO	8 mg/kg/day if <50 kg (adults 400 mg/day) (I) For convalescent oral therapy of serious infections, up to 20 mg/kg/day (III)	q12-24h
Cefotaxime*, Claforan	0.5-, 1-, 2-, 10-g vial	IV, IM	50–180 mg/kg/day (adults 3–8 g/day) (I)	q6-8h
			200–225 mg/kg/day for meningitis (adults 12 g/day) (I)	q6-8h
Cefotetan*, Cefotan	1-, 2-, 10-g vial 1-, 2-g ivpb	IV, IM	60–100 mg/kg/day (II)	q12h
			Adults 2–4 g/day (I)	q12h
Cefoxitin*, Mefoxin	1-, 2-, 10-g vial, 1-, 2-g ivpb	IV, IM	80–160 mg/kg/day, max 12 g/day (I)	q6h
Cefpodoxime*, Vantin	50-, 100-mg/5-mL susp 100-, 200-mg tab	PO	10 mg/kg/day, max 400 mg/day (I)	q12h
Cefprozil*. Cefzil	125-, 250-mg/5-mL susp 250-, 500-mg tab	PO	15–30 mg/kg/day (adults 0.5–1 g/day) (I)	q12h
Ceftazidime*, Ceptaz, Fortaz	0.5-, 1-, 2-, 6-g vial	IV, IM	90–150 mg/kg/day (adults 3–6 g/day) (I)	q8h
	1-, 2-g ivpb		200–300 mg/kg/day for serious Pseudomonas infection (III)	q8h

A. SYSTEMIC ANTIMICROBIALS WITH DOSAGE FORMS AND USUAL DOSAGES (cont)

Generic and Trade Names	Dosage Form	Route	Dose (evidence grade)	Interval
Ceftibuten, Cedax	90-, 180-mg/5-mL susp 400-mg cap	PO	9 mg/kg/day (adults 400 mg/day) (I)	q24h
Ceftizoxime, Cefizox	1-, 2-g/50-mL ivpb	IV, IM	150-200 mg/kg/day (adults 2-12 g/day) (I)	q6-8h
Ceftriaxone*, Rocephin	0.25-, 0.5-, 1-, 2-, 10-g vial 1-, 2-g ivpb	IV, IM	50-75 mg/kg/day, max 2 g/day (I) 100 mg/kg/day for meningitis, max 4 g/day (I) 50 mg/kg for 1-3 doses IM for AOM, max 1 g (II)	q12-24h
Cefuroxime axetil*, Ceftin	125-, 250-mg/5-mL susp 250-, 500-mg tab	PO	20-30 mg/kg/day (adults 0.5-1 g/day) (I) For bone and joint infections, up to 100 mg/kg/day (III)	q12h
Cefuroxime sodium*, Zinacef	0.75-, 1.5-g vial, ivpb	IV, IM	100-150 mg/kg/day (adults 1.5-3 g/day) (I)	q8h
Cephalexin*, Keflex	125-, 250-mg/5-mL susp 125-, 250-mg dispersible tab 250-, 500-mg caps and tabs	PO	25-50 mg/kg/day, max 1 g/day (I) 75-100 mg/kg/day for bone and joint, or severe infections (II) Adults 2-4 g/day (I)	q12h q6h
Chloramphenicol sodium succinate*, Chloromycetin	1-g vial	IV	50-75 mg/kg/day 75-100 mg/kg/day for meningitis (I) Adults max 100 mg/kg/day	q6h
Chloroquine phosphate*, Aralen	250-, 500-mg (150-, 300-mg base) tabs	PO	See Chapter 10.	
Ciprofloxacin*, Cipro	250-, 500-mg/5-mL susp 100-, 250-, 500-, 750-mg tab	PO	20-40 mg/kg/day, max 1.5 g/day (I)	q12h
	200-, 400-mg vial, ivpb	IV	20-30 mg/kg/day, max 1.2 g/day (I)	q8-12h
Ciprofloxacin extended release*,	500-, 1,000-mg ER tab	PO	Adults 500-1,000 mg (I)	q24h

Drug	Formulation	Dose	Route	Interval
Clarithromycin*, Biaxin	125-, 250-mg/5-mL susp 250-, 500-mg tab	15 mg/kg/day, max 1 g/day (I)	PO	q12h
Clarithromycin extended release*, Biaxin XL*	500-mg ER tab	Adults 1,000 mg (I)	PO	q24h
Clindamycin*, Cleocin	75 mg/5-mL soln 75-, 150-, 300-mg cap	10–25 mg/kg/day (adults 1.2–1.8 g/day) (I) 30–40 mg/kg/day for CA-MRSA, intra-abdominal infection, or AOM (III)	PO	q8h
	0.3-, 0.6-, 0.9-g vial, ivpb	20–40 mg/kg/day (adults 1.8–2.7 g/day) (I)	IV, IM	q8h
Clotrimazole*, Mycelex	10-mg lozenge	≥3 y and adults, dissolve lozenge in mouth (I)	PO	5 times daily
Colistimethate*, Coly-Mycin M	150-mg (colistin base) vial	2.5–5 mg/kg/day based on IBW (I) up to 5–7 mg/kg/day (III)	IV, IM	q8h
Cycloserine*, Seromycin	250-mg cap	10–20 mg/kg/day (III) Adults max 1 g/day (I)	PO	q12h
Dapsone*	25-, 100-mg tab	2 mg/kg, max 100 mg (II)	PO	q24h
Daptomycin, Cubicin	500-mg vial	2–5 y 10 mg/kg (III) ≥6–11 y 7 mg/kg (II) ≥12 y and adults 4–6 mg/kg TBW (I)	IV	q24h
Darunavir, Prezista	75-, 150-, 300-, 400-, 600-mg tab	≥ 6 y of age (I): ≥20–<30 kg: 375 mg + ritonavir 50 mg ≥30–<40 kg: 450 mg + ritonavir 60 mg ≥40 kg: 600 mg + ritonavir 100 mg	PO	q12h
Delavirdine, Rescriptor	100-, 200-mg tab	≥16 y 1,200 mg/day (I)	PO	q8h
Demeclocycline*, Declomycin	150-, 300-mg tab	≥8 y 7–13 mg/kg/day, max 600 mg/day (I)	PO	q6h

A. SYSTEMIC ANTIMICROBIALS WITH DOSAGE FORMS AND USUAL DOSAGES (cont)

Generic and Trade Names	Dosage Form	Route	Dose (evidence grade)	Interval
Dicloxacillin*, Dynapen	250-, 500-mg cap	PO	12–25 mg/kg/day (adults 0.5–1 g/day) (I) For bone and joint infections, up to 100 mg/kg/day (III)	q6h
Didanosine (ddI), Videx	50-mg/5-mL oral soln	PO	2 wk–3 mo 50-100 mg/m² (II) >3–8 mo 100 mg/m² (II) >8 mo 90–150 mg/m² (max 200 mg) (I)	q12h
Videx-EC*	125-, 200-, 250-, 400-mg cap	PO	20–<25 kg: 200 mg, 25–<60 kg: 250 mg, ≥60 kg: 400 mg (I)	q24h
Diiodohydroxyquin (see Iodoquinol)				
Doxycycline*	50-, 75-, 100-mg cap, tab 50-mg/5-mL susp	PO	≥8 y, ≤45 kg: 2–4 mg/kg/day (adults 100–200 mg/day) (I)	q12h
	100-mg vial	IV		
Efavirenz, Sustiva	50-, 200-mg cap, 600-mg tab	PO	367 mg/m² max 600 mg (III) ≥ 3 y (I): 10–<15 kg: 200 mg 15–<20 kg: 250 mg 20–<25 kg: 300 mg 25–<32.5 kg: 350 mg 32.5–<40 kg: 400 mg ≥40 kg: 600 mg Adults 600 mg (I)	q24h
Atripla	Combination tab with 200 mg emtricitabine, 300 mg tenofovir, 600 mg efavirenz	PO	Adults 1 tab (I)	q24h
Emtricitabine, Emtriva	50-mg/5-mL soln 200-mg cap	PO	0–3 mo 3mg/kg (I) ≥3 mo: 6 mg/kg, max 240-mg soln (I) >33 kg and adults 200-mg cap (I)	q24h

Truvada	Combination tab with 200 mg emtricitabine + 300 mg tenofovir	PO	Adults 1 tab (I)	q24h
Atripla	Combination tab with 200 mg emtricitabine, 300 mg tenofovir, 600 mg efavirenz	PO	Adults 1 tab (I)	q24h
Enfuvirtide, Fuzeon	108-mg vial (90 mg/mL)	SQ	≥6 y: 2 mg/kg, max 90 mg (I)	q12h
Ertapenem, Invanz	1-g vial	IV, IM	30 mg/kg/day, max 1 g/day (I) ≥13 y and adults 1 g/day (I)	q12h q24h
Erythromycin* base	250-, 500-mg tab, film coated	PO	50 mg/kg/day (adults 1–4 g/day) (I)	q6–8h
Erythromycin coated pellets*, ERYC	250-mg cap, EC			
Erythromycin coated base, PCE	333-, 500-mg tabs of EC particles			
Erythromycin delayed release*, Ery-Tab	250-, 333-, 500-mg tab, EC			
Erythromycin ethylsuccinate*, EES, EryPed	200-, 400-mg/5-mL susp	PO	50 mg/kg/day (adults 1–4 g/day) (I)	q6–8h
Erythromycin ethylsuccinate and sulfisoxazole acetyl*, Pediazole	200 mg erythromycin and 600 mg sulfisoxazole/5-mL susp	PO	50 mg/kg/day of erythromycin component, max 2 g/day erythromycin (I)	q6–8h
Erythromycin lactobionate*, Erythrocin	0.5-, 1-g vial	IV	20 mg/kg/day (adults 1–4 g/day) (I)	q6h
Erythromycin stearate*	250-mg tab, film coated	PO	50 mg/kg/day (adults 1–4 g/day) (I)	q6–8h
Ethambutol*, Myambutol	100-, 400-mg tab	PO	15–25 mg/kg, max 2.5 g (I)	q24h
Ethionamide*, Trecator	250-mg tab	PO	15–20 mg/kg/day, max 1 g/day (III)	q12h

A. SYSTEMIC ANTIMICROBIALS WITH DOSAGE FORMS AND USUAL DOSAGES (cont)

Generic and Trade Names	Dosage Form	Route	Dose (evidence grade)	Interval
Famciclovir*, Famvir	125-, 250-, 500-mg tab	PO	Adults 0.5–1.5 g/day (I)	q8–12h
Fluconazole*, Diflucan	50-, 100-, 150-, 200-mg tab 50-, 200-mg/5-mL susp	PO	3–12 mg/kg/day, max 600 mg/day (I) Max doses 800–1,000 mg/day may be used for some CNS fungal infections (II,III)	q24h q12h for PO high dose
	200-, 400-mg vial, ivpb	IV		
Flucytosine, Ancobon	250-, 500-mg cap	PO	50–150 mg/kg/day (III)	q6h
Fosamprenavir, Lexiva	250-mg/5-mL susp 700-mg tab	PO	≥2 y 60 mg/kg/day, max 2.8 g/day (I) ≥6 y 36 mg/kg/day, max 1,400 mg/day, if boosted with ritonavir 6 mg/kg/day (I)	q12h
Foscarnet*, Foscavir	6-, 12-g vial	IV	CMV/VZV: 180 mg/kg/day (I)	q8h
			CMV suppression: 90–120 mg/kg (I)	q24h
			HSV: 120 mg/kg/day (I)	q8–12h
Ganciclovir*, Cytovene	500-mg vial	IV	CMV treatment: 10–15 mg/kg/day (I)	q12h
			CMV suppression: 5 mg/kg (I)	q24h
			VZV: 10 mg/kg/day (III)	q12h
	250-, 500-mg cap	PO	90 mg/kg/day (III) Adults 3 g/day (I)	q8h
Gemifloxacin, Factive	320-mg tab	PO	Adults 320 mg (I)	q24h
Gentamicin*	20-mg/2-mL pediatric vial 80-mg/2-mL, 800-mg/20-mL adult vial, numerous ivpb	IV, IM	3–7.5 mg/kg/day (cystic fibrosis 7–10); see Chapter 1 regarding q24h dosing	q8–24h
Griseofulvin microsized*, Grifulvin V	125-mg/5-mL susp 500-mg tab	PO	15–25 mg/kg (III) Adults 0.5–1 g (I)	q24h

Drug	Formulation	Route	Dosage	Frequency
Griseofulvin ultramicrosized*, Gris-PEG	125-, 250-mg tab	PO	10–15 mg/kg (III) Adults 0.375–0.75 g (I)	q24h
Imipenem/cilastatin, Primaxin	250/250-, 500/500-mg vial for IV 500/500-mg vial for IM	IV IM	60–100 mg/kg/day (I) IM form not approved for <12 y	q6h
Iodoquinol*, Yodoxin	210-, 650-mg tab	PO	30–40 mg/kg/day, max 1.95 g/day (I)	q8h
Isoniazid*, Nydrazid	50-mg/5-mL syrup 100-, 300-mg tab 1,000-mg vial	PO, IV, IM	10–15 mg/kg/day, max 300 mg/day (I) With directly observed biweekly therapy, dosage is 20–30 mg/kg, max 900 mg/dose (I)	q12–24h Twice weekly
Itraconazole*, Sporanox	50-mg/5-mL soln 100-mg cap*	PO	5 mg/kg/day (I) For serious infections, up to 10 mg/kg/day (III)	q12h
	250-mg vial	IV	5 mg/kg/day (II)	q12h
Ivermectin, Stromectol	3-mg tab	PO	150–200 µg/kg (I)	1 dose
Ketoconazole*, Nizoral	200-mg tab	PO	≥2 y 3.3–6.6 mg/kg/day (II)	q24h
Lamivudine, Epivir	50-mg/5-mL soln 150-, 300-mg tab	PO	Neonates (<30 days): 4 mg/kg/day Infants/children: 8 mg/kg/day max 300 mg/day Adolescents/adults (≥16 y; ≥50 kg): 150 mg/dose q12h or 300 mg once daily (I)	q12h
Epivir HBV	100-mg tab, 25-mg/5-mL soln	PO	3 mg/kg (max 100 mg)	q24h
Combivir	Combination tab: 300 mg zidovudine + 150 mg lamivudine		>12 y and adults 1 tab/dose	q12h
Epzicom	Combination tab with 600 mg abacavir – 300 mg lamivudine		Adults 1 tab	q24h
Trizivir	Combination tab with 300 mg abacavir, 300 mg zidovudine, 150 mg lamivudine		Adults >40 kg 1 tab/dose	q12h

A. SYSTEMIC ANTIMICROBIALS WITH DOSAGE FORMS AND USUAL DOSAGES (cont)

Generic and Trade Names	Dosage Form	Route	Dose (evidence grade)	Interval
Levofloxacin*, Levaquin	125-mg/5-mL soln 250-, 500-, 750-mg tab, 500-, 750-mg vial 250-, 500-, 750-mg ivpb	PO, IV	16 mg/kg/day div q12h up to 50 kg body weight, then 500 mg qd for post-exposure anthrax prophylaxis (I) For respiratory infections <5 y 20 mg/kg/day (II) ≥5 y 10 mg/kg/day (II)	q12h q12h q24h
Linezolid, Zyvox	100-mg/5-mL susp 600-mg tab 200-, 600-mg ivpb		30 mg/kg/day (I) ≥12 y, adults 1,200 mg/day (I)	q8h q12h
Lopinavir/ritonavir, Kaletra – adjustments necessary for concomitant use with nevirapine or efavirenz	400 mg lopinavir/100 mg ritonavir per 5-mL oral soln 100/25-mg pediatric tab 200/50-mg adult tab	PO	≤12 mo: 32 mg/kg/day L (lopinavir) (I) >12 mo, <15 kg: 24 mg/kg/day L (I) 15–<40 kg 20 mg/kg/day L (I) ≥40 kg 800 mg/day L (adult dose) (I)	q12h
Maraviroc (Selzentry)	150-, 300-mg tab	PO	Adolescents ≥16 y/adults: 300–1,200 mg/day (depends on coadministered drugs) (I)	q12h
Mebendazole*, Vermox	100-mg chewable tab	PO	See Chapter 10 for parasite-specific recommendations.	
Mefloquine*, Lariam	250-mg tab	PO	See Chapter 10 for detailed weight-based recommendations for malaria.	
Meropenem*, Merrem	0.5-, 1-g vial	IV	60 mg/kg/day, max 3 g/day (I) 120 mg/kg/day meningitis, max 6 g/day (I)	q8h q8h
Methenamine hippurate*, Hiprex	1-g tab	PO	6–12 y 1–2 g/day (I) >12 y 2 g/day (I)	q12h

Metronidazole*, Flagyl	250-, 500-mg tab, 375-mg cap	PC	30–50 mg/kg/day (adults 750–2250 mg/day) (I)	q8h
	500-mg vial, ivpb	IV	22.5–40 mg/kg/day (II) Adults 1,500 mg/day (I)	q8h
Micafungin*, Mycamine	50-, 100-mg vial	IV	2–4 mg/kg, max 200 mg (I)	q24h
Miconazole*, Oravig	50-mg buccal tab	PO	≥16 y and adults: 50 mg buccal tab	q24h
Minocycline*, Minocin	50-, 75-, 100-mg cap, tab 100-mg vial	PO IV	≥8 y 4 mg/kg/day (adults 200 mg/day) (I)	q12h
Minocycline, extended release*, Solodyn	45-, 90-, 135-mg ER tab	PO	≥12 y 1 mg/kg/day (acne) (I)	q24h
Moxifloxacin, Avelox	400-mg tab 400-mg ivpb	PO, IV	Adults 400 mg/day (I)	q24h
Nafcillin*, Nallpen	1-, 2-, 10-g vial, 1-, 2-g ivpb	IV, IM	150–200 mg/kg/day (II) Adults 3–6 g/day q4h (I)	q6h
Nelfinavir, Viracept	250-, 625-mg tab	PO	>2 y 90–110 mg/kg/day max 2.5 g/day (I)	q12h
Neomycin sulfate*, Neo-fradin	500-mg tab 125-mg/5-mL soln	PO	50–100 mg/kg/day (II)	q6–8h
Nevirapine, Viramune	50-mg/5-mL susp, 200-mg tab	PO	<8 y: 400 mg/m²/day (I) ≥8 y: 240–300 mg/m²/day max 400 mg/day (I) Initiate with half dose once daily for 14 days (I)	q12h
Nitazoxanide, Alinia	500-mg tab; 100-mg/5-mL susp	PO	1–3 y: 200 mg/day 4–11 y: 400 mg/day ≥12 y: 1 g/day (I)	q12h
Nitrofurantoin*, Furadantin	25-mg/5-mL susp	PO	5–7 mg/kg/day 1–2 mg/kg once daily for UTI prophylaxis (I)	q6h
Nitrofurantoin, macrocrystalline*, Macrodantin	25-, 50-, 100-mg cap		5–7 mg/kg/day 1–2 mg/kg once daily for UTI prophylaxis (I)	q6h

A. SYSTEMIC ANTIMICROBIALS WITH DOSAGE FORMS AND USUAL DOSAGES (cont)

Generic and Trade Names	Dosage Form	Route	Dose (evidence grade)	Interval
Nitrofurantoin monohydrate and macrocrystalline*, Macrobid	100-mg cap		>12 y 200 mg/day (I)	q12h
Norfloxacin, Noroxin	400-mg tab	PO	Adults 800 mg/day (I)	q12h
Nystatin*, Mycostatin	500,000-unit/5-mL susp	PO	Infants 2 mL/dose, children 4–6 mL/dose, to coat oral mucosa	q6h
Oseltamivir, Tamiflu	30-mg/5-mL susp 30-, 45-, 75-mg cap	PO	Term infants, birth to 12 mo: 6 mg/kg/day (II). Insufficient data to recommend a dose for premature infants. ≥1 y and ≤15 kg: 60 mg/day (I) >15–23 kg: 90 mg/day (I) >23–40 kg: 120 mg/day (I) >40 kg: 150 mg/day (I)	q12h
			Prophylaxis: give 1/2 daily treatment dose	q24h
Oxacillin* Bactocill	250-, 500-mg, 1-, 2-, 10-g vial	IV, IM	100 mg/kg/day (adults 4–12 g/day) (I) 150–200 mg/kg/day for meningitis (III)	q4–6h
Palivizumab, Synagis	50-, 100-mg vial	IM	15 mg/kg (I)	Monthly
Paromomycin*, Humatin	250-mg cap	PO	25–35 mg/kg/day (adult max 4 g/day) (I)	q8h
Penicillin G benzathine*, Bicillin L-A	600,000 units/mL in 1-, 2-, 4-mL syringe sizes	IM	50,000 units/kg for newborns and infants children <60 lbs 300,000–600,000 units children ≥60 lbs 900,000 units (I) (First FDA-approved in 1952 for dosing by pounds body weight)	1 dose for treatment

Penicillin G benzathine/ procaine*, Bicillin C-R	600,000 units/mL as 300,000 units benzathine + 300,000 units procaine per mL ir 2-mL syringe size	IM	<30 lbs 500,000 units 30–60 lbs 900,000–1,200,000 units >60 lbs 2,400,000 units (I)	1 dose usually (may need repeat injections q 2–3 days
Penicillin G procaine*	600,000 un ts/mL in 1-, 2-mL syringe sizes	IM	50,000 units/kg/day, max 1,200,000 units per dose (I)	q12–24h
Penicillin G K*, Pfizerpen	5-, 20-million unit vial 1-, 2-, 3-million unit IVPB	IV, IM	100,000–250,000 units/kg/day (I)	q4–6h
Penicillin G sodium*	5-million unit vial			
Penicillin V K*	125-, 250-mg/5-mL soln 250-, 500-mg tab	PO	25–50 mg/kg/day (I)	q6h
Pentamidine*, Pentam	300-mg vial	IV, IM	4 mg/kg/day (I)	q24h
Nebupent	300-mg vial	Inhaled	300 mg q month for prophylaxis (I)	q24h
Piperacillin/ tazobactam*, Zosyn	2/0.25-, 3/0.375-, 4/0.5-g vial 36/4.5-g vial	IV	≤40 kg: 240–300 mg PIP/kg/day (adults 12–16 g PIP/day q6h) (I)	q8h
Posaconazole, Noxafil	200-mg/5-mL susp	PO	≥13 y and adults (I): 100 mg q12h for 2 doses then 100 mg/day for oropharyngeal candidiasis (OPC) 600 mg/day for prophylaxis 800 mg/day for refractory OPC	q24h q8h q12h
Praziquantel, Biltricide	600-mg triscored tab	PO	20–25 mg/kg q4–6h for 3 doses (I)	
Primaquine phosphate*	(15-mg base) tab	PO	0.3 mg (base)/kg for PCP, max 30 mg/day (with clindamycin). (III) See also Chapter 10.	q24h
Pyrantel*	250-mg chew tab 250-mg/5-mL susp		11 mg/kg, max 1 g (I)	Once

A. SYSTEMIC ANTIMICROBIALS WITH DOSAGE FORMS AND USUAL DOSAGES (cont)

Generic and Trade Names	Dosage Form	Route	Dose (evidence grade)	Interval
Pyrazinamide*	500-mg tab	PO	15–30 mg/kg/day, max 2 g/day (I)	q24h
			Directly observed biweekly therapy, 40–50 mg/kg (I)	Twice weekly
Quinupristin/ dalfopristin Synercid	150/350-mg vial (500 mg total)	IV	22.5 mg/kg/day (II) Adults 15–22.5 mg/kg/day (I)	q8h q8–12h
Raltegravir, Isentress	400-mg tab	PO	>6 y, >25 kg 800 mg/day (II) ≥16 y and adults 800 mg/day (I)	q12h
Ribavirin*, Rebetol	200-mg cap/tab 400-, 600-mg tab 200-mg/5-mL soln	PO	15 mg/kg/day (with interferon 3 times/week) (III)	q12h
Ribavirin, inhalation*, Virazole	6-g vial	Inhaled	1 vial by SPAG-2	q24h
Rifabutin, Mycobutin	150-mg cap	PO	5 mg/kg for MAC prophylaxis (II) 10–20 mg/kg for MAC or TB treatment (I) Max 300 mg/day	q24h
Rifampin*, Rifadin	150-, 300-mg cap, 600-mg vial	PO, IV	10–20 mg/kg, max 600 mg for TB (I)	q24h
			With directly observed biweekly therapy, dosage is still 10–20 mg/kg/dose (max 600 mg)	Twice weekly
			20 mg/kg/day for 2 days for meningococcus prophylaxis, adult dose 1,200 mg/day (I)	q12h
Rifampin/Isoniazid*, Rifamate	300/150-mg cap	PO	Refer to individual agents.	
Rifampin/isoniazid/ pyrazinamide, Rifater	120/50/300-mg tab	PO	Refer to individual agents.	

				Twice weekly
Rifapentine, Priftin	150-mg tab	PO	≥12 y and adults: 600 mg/dose (I)	
Rifaximin, Xifaxan	200-mg tab	PO	≥12 y and adults: 600 mg/day (I)	q8h
Rimantadine*, Flumadine	100-mg tab	PO	≥1 y, 5 mg/kg/day, max 150 mg/day (III) ≥10 y and adults, 200 mg/day (I)	q12h q12h
Ritonavir, Norvir	100-mg cap, tab 400-mg/5-mL soln		As pharmacokinetic enhancer of other HIV protease inhibitors: 3–12 mg/kg/day (I)	q12h
Saquinavir, Invirase	200-mg hard gel cap 500-mg tab	PO	≥2 y 100 mg/kg/day + ritonavir 5–6 mg/kg/day (II) Adolescent/adults 2,000 mg/day + ritonavir 200 mg/day (I)	q12h
Stavudine*, Zerit	5-mg/5-mL soln 15-, 20-, 30-, 40-mg cap	PO	Birth–13 days of age 1 mg/kg/day (I) ≥14 days, <30 kg 2 mg/kg/day (I) 30–<60 kg: 60 mg/day (I) ≥60 kg: 80 mg/day (I)	q12h
Streptomycin*	1-g vial	IM, IV	20–30 mg/kg/day, max 1 g/day (I)	q12h
Sulfadiazine*	500-mg tab	PO	120–150 mg/kg/day, max 4–6 g/day (I)	q6h
			Rheumatic fever secondary prophylaxis 500 mg once daily if ≤27 kg 1,000 mg once daily if >27 kg (II)	q24h
			See also Chapter 10.	
Telbivudine, Tyzeka	600-mg tab	PO	≥16 y and adults 600 mg/day	q24h
Telithromycin, Ketek	300-, 400-mg tab	PO	Adults 800 mg/day (I)	q24h
Tenofovir, Viread	300-mg tab	PO	≥12 y and adults 300 mg (I)	q24h
Truvada	Combination tab with 200 mg emtricitabine + 300 mg tenofovir	PO	Adults 1 tab	q24h
Atripla	Combination tab with 200 mg emtricitabine, 300 mg tenofovir, 600 mg efavirenz	PO	Adults 1 tab	q24h

A. SYSTEMIC ANTIMICROBIALS WITH DOSAGE FORMS AND USUAL DOSAGES (cont)

Generic and Trade Names	Dosage Form	Route	Dose (evidence grade)	Interval
Terbinafine*, Lamisil	125-, 187.5-mg oral granules 250-mg tab*	PO	>4 y <25 kg 125 mg/day, 25–35 kg 187.5 mg/day, >35 kg 250 mg/day (I)	q24h
Tetracycline*	250-, 500-mg cap, tab	PO	≥8 y 25–50 mg/kg/day (I)	q6h
Ticarcillin/clavulanate, Timentin	3/0.1-g vial, ivpb, 30/1-g vial	IV	200–300 mg ticarcillin/kg/day (adults 12–18 g/day) (I)	q4–6h
Tinidazole, Tindamax	250-, 500-mg tab	PO	50 mg/kg, max 2 g (I) See also Chapter 10.	q24h
Tipranavir, Aptivus	500-mg/5-mL soln, 250-mg cap	PO	≥2 y: 28 mg/kg/day + ritonavir 12 mg/kg/day (adults 1,000 mg/day + ritonavir 400 mg/day) (I)	q12h
Tobramycin*, Nebcin	20-mg/2-mL pediatric vial 80-mg/2-mL, 1.2-g vial	IV, IM	3–7.5 mg/kg/day (cystic fibrosis 7–10); see Chapter 1 regarding q24h dosing	q8–24h
Tobraycin, inhalation, Tobi	300-mg ampule	Inhaled	≥6 y 600 mg/day	q12h
Trimethoprim/ sulfamethoxazole*, Bactrim, Septra	80-mg TMP/400-mg SMX tab (single strength) 160-mg TMP/800-mg SMX tab (double strength) 40-mg TMP/200-mg SMX per 5-mL susp 16-mg TMP/80-mg SMX per mL inj soln in 5-, 10-, 30-mL vials	PO, IV	8–10 mg TMP/kg/day (I)	q12h
			2 mg TMP/kg/day for UTI prophylaxis (I)	q24h
			15–20 mg TMP/kg/day for PCP treatment (I)	q6–8h
			150 mg TMP/m²/day div bid, 3 times each week for PCP prophylaxis (I)	3 times a week
Valacyclovir*, Valtrex	500-mg, 1-g tab	PO	VZV: ≥3 mo, 60 mg/kg/day (I,II) HSV: ≥3 mo, 40 mg/kg/day (II) Max single dose 1 g (I)	q8h q12h

Drug	Formulations	Route	Dose	Interval
Valganciclovir, Valcyte	250-mg/5-mL susp, 450-mg tab	PO	CMV treatment: 32 mg/kg/day (II); CMV prophylaxis: 7 x BSA x CrCl (using the modified Schwartz formula for CrCl, see Chapter 14) Max 900 mg (I)	q12h q24h
			Adults 900–1,800 mg/day (I)	q12–24h
Vancomycin*, Vancocin	125-, 250-mg cap	PO	40 mg/kg/day (I), max 500 mg/day (III)	q6h
	0.5-, 0.75-, 1-, 5-, 10-g vial*; 0.5-, 0.75-, 1-g ivpb	IV	30–40 mg/kg/day (adjusted based on therapeutic drug monitoring) (I) For life-threatening invasive MRSA infection, 60 mg/kg/day to achieve trough serum concentrations above 15 µg/mL (III)	q6–8h
Voriconazole, Vfend	200-mg/5-mL susp, 50-, 200-mg tab, 200-mg vial	IV, PO	Aspergillosis: 12–16 mg/kg/day (IV) or 18 mg/kg/day (PO) loading dose (max 800 mg/day) x 1 day, then 16 mg/kg/day (max 400 mg/day) (I); see also Section VI Adults 200–400 mg/day (I)	q12h
Zanamivir, Relenza	5-mg blister cap for inhalation	Inhaled	Prophylaxis: ≥5 y 10 mg (I)	q24h
			Treatment: ≥7 y 10 mg (I)	q12h
Zidovudine, Retrovir	50-mg/5-mL syrup*, 100-mg cap*, 300-mg tab*, 200-mg/20-mL vial	PO	4–<9 kg 24 mg/kg/day, 9–<30 kg 18 mg/kg/day, ≥30 kg and adults 600 mg/day (I) Cr 480 mg/m²/day (max 600 mg/day) (I)	q12h
		IV	480 mg/m²/day (max 600 mg/day) (II) 20 mg/m²/hour continuous infusion (II)	q6h
Combivir	Combination tab: 300 mg zidovudine		>12 y and adults 1 tab/dose (I) + 150 mg lamivudine	q12h
Trizivir	Combination tab with 300 mg abacavir, 300 mg zidovudine, lamivudine		Adults 1 tab/dose (I)	q12h

* Available in a generic formulation.

B. TOPICAL ANTIMICROBIALS (SKIN, EYE, EAR)

Generic and Trade Names	Dosage Form	Route	Dose (evidence grade)	Interval
Acyclovir, Zovirax	5% cream	Top	≥12 y apply to oral lesion	5 times a day
	5% oint[a]		Apply to genital lesion	6 times a day
Azithromycin, AzaSite	1% ophth soln	Ophth	1 gtt	bid for 2 days then daily for 5 days
Bacitracin	ophth oint	Ophth	Apply to affected eye.	q3–4h
	oint[b,c]	Top	Apply to affected area.	bid–qid
Besifloxacin, Besivance	0.6% ophth susp	Ophth	≥1 y 1 gtt to affected eye	tid
Butenafine, Mentax	1% cream	Top	≥12 y apply to affected area	qd
Butoconazole[a], Gynazole-1	2% cream	Vag	Insert intravaginally	qd for 1 day
Femstat-3				qd for 3 days
Chloramphenicol, Chloromycetin	1% ophth oint	Ophth	Apply to affected eye	q3h
Ciclopirox[b], Loprox	0.77% cream, gel, lotion	Top	≥10 y apply to affected area	bid
	1% shampoo[a]			q3–4 d
	8% nail lacquer[a]			qd
Ciprofloxacin, Ciloxan	0.3% ophth soln[b]	Ophth	≥12 y apply to affected eye	q2h for 2 days then q4h for 5 days
	0.3% ophth oint[a]			q8h for 2 days then q12h for 5 days

Drug	Formulation	Route	Instructions	Frequency
Ciprofloxacin, Cetraxal Cipro HC (plus hydrocortisone) Otic	0.2% otic soln	Otic	≥1 y apply 3 drops to affected ear	bid for 7 days
Ciprofloxacin + dexamethasone, Ciprodex	0.3% otic soln	Otic	≥6 mo apply 4 drops to affected ear	bid for 7 days
Clindamycin, Clindesse	2% cream	Vag	Adolescents 1 applicatorful intravaginally	One time
Cleocin[b]	100-mg supp		1 supp intravaginally	qhs for 3 days
	2% cream		1 applicatorful intravaginally	qhs for 3–7 days
Cleocin-T[b]	1% soln, gel, lotion	Top	Apply to affected area	qd–bid
Evoclin	1% foam			qd
Clindamycin + benzoyl peroxide, Benzaclin,	1% gel	Top	≥12 y apply to affected area	bid
Acanya	1.2% gel		Apply small amount to face	q24h
Clindamycin + tretinoin, Ziana, Veltin	1.2% gel	Top	Apply small amount to face	hs
Clotrimazole[a,b,c] Lotrimin	1% cream, lotion, soln	Top	Apply to affected area	bid
Gyne-Lotrimin-7	1% cream, 100-mg supp	Vag	Adolescents intravaginally	qhs for 7–14 days
Gyne-Lotrimin-3	2% cream, 200-mg supp			qhs for 3 days
Clotrimazole + betamethasone, Lotrisone[b]	1% cream, lotion	Top	≥12 y apply to affected area	bid

B. TOPICAL ANTIMICROBIALS (SKIN, EYE, EAR) (cont)

Generic and Trade Names	Dosage Form	Route	Dose (evidence grade)	Interval
Coly-Mycin S Colistin + neomycin + hydrocortisone	otic susp	Otic	Apply 3–4 drops to affected ear canal; may use with wick	q6–8h
Cortisporin x Bacitracin + neomycin + polymyxin b + hydrocortisone	oint[a]	Ophth	Apply to affected eye	q4h
		Top	Apply to affected area	bid–qid
Neomycin + polymyxin b + hydrocortisone	ophth soln[a]	Ophth	1–2 drops to affected eye	q4h
	otic soln, susp	Otic	3 drops to affected ear	tid–qid
	cream[a]	Top	Apply to affected area	
Econazole[b], Spectazole	1% cream	Top	Apply to affected area	bid
Erythromycin	0.5% ophth oint[b]	Ophth	Apply to affected eye	q4h
Eryderm, Erygel	2% soln[b], gel[a,b]	Top	Apply to affected area	bid
Ery Pads	2% pledgets[b]			
Akne-mycin	2% oint			
Erythromycin + benzoyl peroxide, Benzamycin[b]	3% gel	Top	≥12 y apply to affected area	qd–bid
Gatifloxacin, Zymaxid	0.5% ophth soln	Ophth	Apply to affected eye	q2h for 1 day then q6h

Drug	Formulation	Route	Application	Frequency
Gentamicin[b], Garamycin	0.1% cream, oint	Top	Apply to affected area	tid–qid
	0.3% ophth soln, oint	Ophth[a]	Apply to affected eye	q1–4h (sol) q4–8h (oint)
Gentamicin + prednisolone, Pred-G[a]	0.3% ophth soln, oint	Ophth	Apply to affected eye	q1–4h (sol) qd–tid (oint)
Ketoconazole				
Nizoral	shampoo[a,b]	Top	Apply to affected area	qd (for 1 for shampoo)
	2% cream[b]	Top	≥12 y apply to affected area	q3–4 d
Nizoral A-D[c]	1% shampoo	Top	≥12 y apply to affected area	bid
Extina, Xolegel	2% foam, gel	Top	≥12 y apply to affected area	bid
Levofloxacin				
Iquix	1.5% ophth soln	Ophth	Apply to affected eye	q1–4h
Quixin	0.5% ophth soln	Ophth		q1–4h
Mafenide, Sulfamylon	8.5% cream	Top	Apply to burn	qd–bid
	5-g pwd for reconstitution		To keep burn dressing wet	q4–8h as needed
Malathion, Ovide	0.5% soln	Top	≥6 y apply to hair and scalp	Once
Maxitrol[a,3], neomycin + polymyxin b + dexamethasone	susp, oint	Oph-h	Apply to affected eye	q4h (oint) q1–4h (susp)

B. TOPICAL ANTIMICROBIALS (SKIN, EYE, EAR) (cont)

Generic and Trade Names	Dosage Form	Route	Dose (evidence grade)	Interval
Metronidazole[a]				
MetroGel-Vaginal[b]	0.75% vag gel	Vag	1 applicatorful intravaginally	qd–bid
MetroCream-gel,	0.75% cream[b], gel[b], lotion[b]	Top		bid
– lotion				qd
Noritate, MetroGel	1% cream, gel			
Miconazole				
Micatin[b,c] and others	2% cream, pwd, oint, spray, lotion, gel	Top	Apply to affected area	qd–bid
Fungoid[c]	2% tincture			bid
Vusion	0.25% oint		≥1 mo: to diaper dermatitis	Each diaper change for 7 days
Monistat-1	1.2-g vag supp	Vag	Adolescents: Intravaginally	once
Monistat-3[b,c]	4% cream, 200-mg supp			qhs for 3 days
Monistat-7[b,c]	2% cream, 100-mg supp			qhs for 7 days
Moxifloxacin, Vigamox	0.5% ophth soln	Ophth	Apply to affected eye	tid
Mupirocin, Bactroban	2% oint[b], cream, nasal oint	Top	Apply to infected skin or nasal mucosa	tid
Naftifine, Naftin[a]	1% cream, gel	Top	Apply to affected area	Cream qd; gel bid
Natamycin, Natacyn[a]	5% ophth soln	Ophth	Apply to affected eye	q1–4h

Neosporin[b]				
Bacitracin + neomycin	ophth oint[a]	Ophth	Apply to affected eye	q4h
+ polymyxin B	top oint[c]	Top	Apply to affected area	bid–qid
Gramicidin + neomycin + polymyxin B	ophth soln[a]	Ophth	Apply to affected eye	q4h
Nystatin[b], Mycostatin	100,000 units/g cream, oint, pwd	Top	Apply to affected area	bid–qid
	100,000 vag tablet	Vag	Adolescents: intravaginally	qd
Nystatin + triamcinolone 0.1% Mycolog II[b]	100,000 units/g cream, oint	Top	Apply to affected area	bid
Ofloxacin[b], Floxin Otic	0.3% otic soln	Otic	5–10 drops to affected ear	qd–bid
Ocuflox	0.3% ophth soln	Ophth	Apply to affected eye	q1–6h
Oxiconazole, Oxistat	1% cream, lotion	Top	Apply to affected area	qd–bid
Penciclovir, Denavir	1% top cream	Top	Apply to affected area	q2h while awake for 4 days
Permethrin, Nix[b,c]	1% cream	Top	Apply to hair/scalp	Once for 10 min
Elimite[c]	5% cream		Apply to all skin surfaces	Once for 8–14 h
Polysporin[b]	ophth oint[a]	Ophth	Apply to affected eye	q4–6h
polymyxin B + bacitracin	oint[c], pwd[c]	Top	Apply to affected area	
Polytrim[b] trimethoprim + polymyxin B	ophth soln	Ophth	Apply to affected eye	q3–4h

B. TOPICAL ANTIMICROBIALS (SKIN, EYE, EAR) (cont)

Generic and Trade Names	Dosage Form	Route	Dose (evidence grade)	Interval
Pyrethrins[b], Rid	0.3% lotion, gel, shampoo	Top	Apply to affected area	Once for 10 min
Retapamulin, Altabax	1% oint	Top	Apply thin layer to affected area	bid for 5 days
Sertaconazole, Ertaczo	2% cream	Top	Apply to tinea pedis	bid for 4 wk
Silver Sulfadiazine[a,b], Silvadene	1% cream	Top	Apply to affected area	qd–bid
Sulconazole, Exelderm	1% soln, cream	Top	Apply to affected area	qd–bid
Sulfacetamide sodium[b]	10, 15, 30% soln	Ophth	Apply to affected eye	q1–3h qid
Sodium-Sulamyd	10% ophth oint			
Klaron	10% top lotion	Top	≥12 y apply to affected area	bid–qid
Sulfacetamide sodium	10% ophth oint	Ophth	Apply to affected eye	tid–qid
+ prednisolone, Blephamide[b]	10% opth soln			
Sulfacetamide sodium + fluorometholone, FML-S	10% opth soln	Ophth	Apply to affected eye	qid
Terbinafine[c], Lamisil-AT	1% cream[b], spray, gel, soln	Top	Apply to affected area	qd–bid
Terconazole[a,b], Terazol-3	0.4% cream, 80 mg supp			
Terazol-7	0.8% cream	Vag		
Tobramycin[b], Tobrex	0.3% ophth soln, oint	Ophth	Apply to affected eye	q1–4h (sol) q4–8h (oint)

Tobramycin + dexamethasone, Tobradex	0.3% ophth soln[b], oint	Ophth	Apply to affected eye	q2–6h (sol) q6–8h (oint)
Tobramycin + fluorometholone, Tobrasone	0.3% ophth soln[b], oint	Ophth	Apply to affected eye	q2–6h (sol) q6–8h (oint)
Trifluridine[b], Viroptic	1% ophth soln	Ophth	1 drop (max 9 drops/day)	q2h
Tolnaftate, Tinactin	1% cream, soln, pwd, spray	Top	Apply to affected area	bid

[a]Not approved for children.
[b]Generic available.
[c]Over-the-counter.

12. Antibiotic Therapy for Obese Children

The dose of antimicrobial for an obese child that is required to achieve the same tissue site exposure to pathogens as children of average body weight is most often not available. When antimicrobials are first investigated for US Food and Drug Administration approval, obese children are excluded from pharmacokinetic and drug exposure analysis. During the treatment studies required for drug approval, obese children are also excluded, so unless specific studies are performed on this population, no dosing or exposure data exist.

In general, different classes of drugs distribute in a predictable way into different tissue compartments, so a reasonable guess for the proper dose, by class of antibiotic, is possible. For drugs that do not distribute into adipose tissue, dosing should be based on lean body weight. For those that do distribute into adipose tissue, increasing the dose, based on body weight, is logical, although high-dosage regimens may represent an increased risk of toxicity or poor tolerance. For other classes of drugs, distribution into adipose tissue may be intermediate, and the dose should be somewhere in between that calculated for lean body weight and total body weight. For sake of simplicity, dosing guidance by body surface area is not provided.

Listed below are the major classes of antimicrobials and guidance on how to calculate the most appropriate dose. The level of evidence to support these recommendations is Level II–III (based on adult studies). Whenever a dose is used that is greater than one prospectively investigated for efficacy and safety, the clinician must monitor the child closely for unanticipated adverse events. Data are not available on all agents.

Drug Class	Dosing Recommendations		
	By Ideal Body Weight	Intermediate Dosing	By Total Body Weight[a]
ANTIBACTERIALS			
Beta-lactams		IBW + 0.3 (TBW-IBW)	
Penicillins		X	
Cephalosporins		X	
Carbapenems	X		
Macrolides			
Erythromycins	X		
Azithromycin	X (for gastrointestinal infections)		X
Clarithromycin	X		
Lincosamides		IBW + 0.3 (TBW-IBW)	
Clindamycin		X	

Drug Class	Dosing Recommendations		
	By Ideal Body Weight	**Intermediate Dosing**	**By Total Body Weight**[a]
ANTIBACTERIALS (cont)			
Sulfonamide	X		
Glycopeptides			
Vancomycin			X
Aminoglycosides		IBW + 0.4 (TBW-IBW)	
Gentamicin		X	
Tobramycin		X	
Amikacin		X	
Fluoroquinolones		IBW + 0.45 (TBW-IBW)	
Ciprofloxacin		X	
Levofloxacin		X	
Rifamycins			
Rifampin	X		
Miscellaneous			
Metronidazole		IBW + 0.45 (TBW-IBW)	
Linezolid	X		
Daptomycin			X
ANTIFUNGALS			
Amphotericin B (conventional and lipid formulations)			X
Echinocandins			
Caspofungin			X
Micafungin		X	
Azoles			
Fluconazole			X
Voriconazole	X		
Flucytosine	X		

Drug Class	Dosing Recommendations		
	By Ideal Body Weight	Intermediate Dosing	By Total Body Weight[a]
ANTIVIRALS (non-HIV)			
Nucleoside analogues (acyclovir, ganciclovir)	X		
ANTIMYCOBACTERIALS			
Isoniazid	X		
Rifampin	X		
Pyrazinamide	X		
Ethambutol	X		
Streptomycin	X		

Abbreviations: HIV, human immunodeficiency virus; IBW, ideal body weight; TBW, total body weight.
[a] Actual measured body weight.

13. Antibiotic Therapy for Patients With Renal Failure

For anti-infective drugs recently approved by the US Food and Drug Administration (FDA), information on drug exposure in patients with varying degrees of renal failure is placed in the package label and posted on the National Library of Medicine/National Institutes of Health Web site as a collaborative project with the FDA (http://dailymed.nlm.nih.gov/dailymed/about.cfm). Information on older agents is often lacking, and information on children in particular may never have been collected prospectively. A complete list of antibiotics and dosing recommendations in renal failure, and for children on dialysis, is beyond the scope of this chapter. An exhaustive, annually updated reference that includes information on dosing adjustments in renal failure, *AHFS Drug Information 2011,* is available for computer or PDA from the American Society of Hospital Pharmacists, Inc. (http://www.ahfsdruginformation.com/).

Many commonly used antimicrobials are excreted primarily by the kidneys; therefore, when significant renal impairment is present, either downward adjustments in dosages must be made or the intervals between doses must be lengthened. Drugs that are excreted by the kidney and have a narrow therapeutic index, with toxicity documented at serum concentrations not too much greater than therapeutic concentrations, must be monitored closely. The aminoglycosides and vancomycin are prime examples of these antibiotics. For those antibiotics excreted by the kidney, but with little toxicity at high serum concentrations, such as the beta-lactam antibiotics, only moderate changes in dosages need to be made. Drugs such as metronidazole that are metabolized by the liver and those excreted significantly by the liver, such as azithromycin, nafcillin, and ceftriaxone, do not usually require adjustments in dosing in renal failure.

In some circumstances, dosing drugs in children with decreased renal function is best achieved by therapeutic drug monitoring of serum antibiotic concentrations. Many computer programs are available that integrate information on the serum creatinine (or creatinine clearance [CrCl]) and antibiotic half-life, which allows for estimation of the best mg/kg dosage, administered at a specified interval in order to attain therapeutic but nontoxic peak and trough serum concentrations to achieve the most appropriate antibiotic exposure profile for cure (eg, the area under the curve/minimum inhibitory concentration ratio, see Chapter 3). Many hospital-based pharmacists can assist with this determination. The following calculation (commonly known as the modified Schwartz method) is used for estimating CrCl (and therefore antibiotic clearance) in infants and children (1–18 years of age) with stable renal function:

CrCl (mL/min/1.73 m^2 BSA) = (κ x height [cm])/serum creatinine (mg/dL)
BSA = body surface area
κ is a proportionality constant that varies with age and sex:

Preterm infants	0.33
Full-term infants	0.45
Children and adolescent girls	0.55
Adolescent boys	0.78

In the absence of a software program, one can administer the customary initial loading mg/kg dose, and until antibiotic assay results are available, make an estimate of the appropriate dosage based on past experience of rates of excretion related to the degree of renal failure. Alterations in dosage and/or interval are made to achieve serum concentrations and therefore exposure of antibiotic at the site of infection, similar to those in patients with normal renal function.

14. Antimicrobial Prophylaxis/Prevention of Symptomatic Infection

This chapter provides a summary of recommendations for prophylaxis of infections, defined as providing therapy prior to the onset of clinical signs or symptoms of infection. Prophylaxis can be considered in several clinical scenarios.

A. Postexposure Prophylaxis

Given for a short, specified period after exposure to specific pathogens/organisms, where the risks of acquiring the infection are felt to justify antimicrobial treatment to eradicate the pathogen or prevent symptomatic infection in situations in which the child (either healthy or with increased susceptibility to infection) is likely to have been inoculated (eg, asymptomatic child closely exposed to meningococcus, or a neonate born to a mother with active genital HSV).

B. Long-term Symptomatic Disease Prophylaxis

Given to a particular, defined population of children who are of relatively high risk of acquiring a severe infection (eg, a child post-splenectomy, or a child with documented rheumatic heart disease to prevent subsequent streptococcal infection), with prophylaxis provided during the period of risk, potentially months or years.

C. Preemptive Treatment/Latent Infection Treatment ("Prophylaxis of Symptomatic Infection")

Where a child has a documented but asymptomatic infection, and targeted antimicrobials are given to prevent the development of symptomatic disease (eg, latent tuberculosis infection or therapy of a stem cell transplant patient with documented CMV viremia, but no symptoms of infection or rejection). Treatment period is usually defined, but in certain circumstances, such as reactivation of a herpesvirus, may require re-treatment.

D. Surgical/Procedure Prophylaxis

A child receives a surgical/invasive catheter procedure, planned or unplanned, where the risk of infection postoperatively or post-procedure may justify prophylaxis to prevent an infection from occurring (eg, prophylaxis to prevent infection following spinal rod placement). Treatment is usually short-term, beginning just prior to the procedure and ending at the conclusion of the procedure, or within 24 to 48 hours.

E. Travel-Related Exposure Prophylaxis

Not discussed in this chapter; please refer to information on specific disease entities (eg, traveler's diarrhea, Chapter 6) or pathogens (eg, malaria, Chapter 10). Updated, current information for travelers about prophylaxis and current worldwide infection risks can be found on the CDC Web site at http://www.cdc.gov/travel/.

NOTE
- **Abbreviations:** ACOG, American College of Obstetricians and Gynecologists; amox/clav, amoxicillin/clavulanate; bid, twice daily; CDC, Centers for Disease Control and Prevention; CMV, cytomegalovirus; div, divided; GI, gastrointestinal; HSV, herpes simplex virus; IGRA, interferon-gamma release assay; IM, intramuscular; INH, isoniazid; IV, intravenous; MRSA, methicillin-resistant *Staphylococcus aureus;* MRSE, methicillin-resistant *S epidermidis;* PO, orally; PPD, purified protein derivative; qd, once daily; qid, 4 times daily ; TB, tuberculosis; tid, 3 times daily; TIG, tetanus immune globulin; TMP/SMX, trimethoprim/sulfamethoxazole; UTI, urinary tract infection.

A. POSTEXPOSURE PROPHYLAXIS

Prophylaxis Category	Therapy (evidence grade)	Comments
Bacterial		
Bites, animal and human (*Pasteurella multocida* [animal], *Eikenella corrodens* [human], *Staphylococcus* spp and *Streptococcus* spp)	Amox/clav 45 mg/kg/day PO div tid (amox/clav 7:1, see Chapter 1, Aminopenicillins) for 5–10 days (AII) OR ampicillin and clindamycin (BII)	Consider rabies prophylaxis for animal bites (AI); consider tetanus prophylaxis. Human bites have a very high rate of infection (do not close open wounds). *S aureus* coverage is only fair with amox/clav, and provides no coverage for MRSA. For penicillin allergy, consider ciprofloxacin (for *Pasteurella*) plus clindamycin (BIII).

Endocarditis Prophylaxis: Given that (1) endocarditis is rarely caused by dental/GI procedures, and (2) prophylaxis for procedures prevents an exceedingly small number of cases, the risks of antibiotics most often outweigh benefits. However, some "highest risk" conditions are currently recommended for prophylaxis: (1) prosthetic heart valve (or prosthetic material used to repair a valve); (2) previous endocarditis; (3) cyanotic congenital heart disease that is unrepaired (or palliatively repaired with shunts and conduits); (4) congenital heart disease that is repaired but with defects at the site of repair adjacent to prosthetic material; (5) completely repaired congenital heart disease using prosthetic material, for the first 6 months after repair; or (6) cardiac transplant patients with valvulopathy. Routine prophylaxis no longer is required for children with native valve abnormalities.

– In highest risk patients: dental procedures that involve manipulation of the gingival or periodontal region of teeth	Amoxicillin 50 mg/kg PO 1 h before procedure OR ampicillin or ceftriaxone or cefazolin, all at 50 mg/kg IM/IV 30 to 60 min before procedure	If penicillin allergy: clindamycin 20 mg/kg PO (60 min before) or IV (30 min before); OR azithromycin 15 mg/kg or clarithromycin 15 mg/kg, 1 h before
– Genitourinary and gastrointestinal procedures	None	No longer recommended

A. POSTEXPOSURE PROPHYLAXIS (cont)

Prophylaxis Category	Therapy (evidence grade)	Comments
Bacterial (cont)		
Meningococcus (*Neisseria meningitidis*)	For prophylaxis of close family contacts or child care contacts, or for those having contact with respiratory secretions from an infected patient following exposure: Rifampin 10 mg/kg PO q12h for 4 doses OR ceftriaxone 125–250 mg IM once OR ciprofloxacin 500 mg PO once (adolescents and adults)	A few cipro-resistant strains have now been reported.
Pertussis	Azithromycin (10 mg/kg/day for 5 days) or clarithromycin (15 mg/kg/day div bid for 7 days) or erythromycin (estolate preferable) 40 mg/kg/day PO div qid; for 14 days (AII) Alternative: TMP/SMX (8 mg/kg/day TMP) div bid for 14 days (BIII)	Prophylaxis to family members and close contacts Azithromycin and clarithromycin are better tolerated than erythromycin (Chapter 5); azithromycin is preferred in exposed young infants, to reduce pyloric stenosis risk.
Tetanus (*Clostridium tetani*)	TIG 250 U IM, once, for those with <3 tetanus immunizations (AII). For deep, contaminated wounds, wound debridement essential. For wounds that cannot be fully debrided, consider metronidazole 30 mg/kg/day PO div q8h until wound healing is underway, and anaerobic conditions no longer exist, as short as 3–5 days (BII).	Immunize with Td, DTaP, or Tdap if not current.
Tuberculosis (*Mycobacterium tuberculosis*) Exposed infant <4 y, or immunocompromised patient (high risk of dissemination)	Exposed infant <4 y, or immunocompromised patient (high risk of dissemination): INH 10–15 mg/kg PO daily for 2–3 mo after last exposure with repeat skin test or IGRA test negative (AIII)	If PPD or IGRA remains negative at 2–3 mo and child remains well, consider stopping empiric therapy. However, tests at 2–3 mo may not be reliable in immunocompromised patients.

Viral		
Herpes Simplex Virus		
During pregnancy	For women with recurrent genital herpes: acyclovir 400 mg PO bid; valacyclovir 500 mg PO qd OR 1 g PO qd from 36 wk gestation until delivery (CII)	ACOG recommends maternal antiviral prophylaxis in HSV-2 seropositive women. Development of neonatal HSV disease after maternal suppression has been documented.
Neonatal	300 mg/m²/dose PO tid for 6 mo following cessation of IV acyclovir treatment of acute disease (AI)	Follow absolute neutrophil counts at 2 and 4 wk, then monthly during prophylactic/suppressive therapy
Keratitis (ocular)	300 mg/m²/dose PO tid for 12 mo following cessation of treatment of acute disease (AII)	Based on data from adults. Watch for severe recurrence at conclusion of suppression.
Influenza virus (A or B)	Oseltamivir Based on body weight for children >12 mo ≤15 kg: 30 mg qd >15–23 kg: 45 mg qd >23–40 kg: 60 mg qd >40 kg: 75 mg qd Infants 3–<12 mo: 3 mg/kg per dose qd Infants 0–≤3 mo: Not recommended unless situation judged critical because of limited data on use in this age group. Zanamivir Children ≥5 y: 10 mg (two 5-mg inhalations) qd	Amantadine and rimantadine are not recommended for prophylaxis.
Rabies virus	Rabies immune globulin, 20 IU/kg, infiltrate around wound, with remaining volume injected IM	Rabies immunization should be provided postexposure.
Fungal		
– *Pneumocystis jiroveci* (previously *Pneumocystis carinii*)	TMP/SMX 5 mg TMP/kg/day PO daily or 3 times/wk (AI); OR dapsone 1 mg/kg PO qd until no longer immunocompromised, based on oncology or transplant treatment regimen	Prophylaxis in specific immunocompromised hosts

B. LONG-TERM SYMPTOMATIC DISEASE PROPHYLAXIS

Prophylaxis Category	Therapy (evidence grade)	Comments
Bacterial otitis media	Amoxicillin or other antibiotics can be used in one-half the therapeutic dose qd or bid to prevent infections if the benefits outweigh the risks of development of resistant organisms for that child.	To prevent recurrent infections, also consider the risks and benefits of placing tympanostomy tubes to improve middle ear ventilation. Studies have demonstrated that amoxicillin, sulfisoxazole, and TMP/SMX are effective. However, antimicrobial prophylaxis may alter the nasopharyngeal flora and foster colonization with resistant organisms, compromising long-term efficacy of the prophylactic drug. Continuous PO-administered antimicrobial prophylaxis should be reserved for control of recurrent acute otitis media, only when defined as ≥3 distinct and well-documented episodes during a period of 6 mo or ≥4 episodes during a period of 12 mo. Although prophylactic administration of an antimicrobial agent limited to a period when a person is at high risk of otitis media has been suggested (eg, during acute viral respiratory tract infection), this method has not been evaluated critically.
Urinary tract infection, recurrent	TMP/SMX (2 mg/kg/dose of TMP) PO qd OR nitrofurantoin 1–2 mg/kg PO qd at bedtime; more rapid resistance may develop using beta-lactams (BII)	Only for those with grade III–V reflux, or with recurrent febrile UTI; prophylaxis no longer recommended for patients with grade I–II (some also exclude grade III) reflux and no evidence of renal damage. Early treatment of new infections is recommended for these children. Resistance eventually develops to every antibiotic; follow resistance patterns for each patient.

C. PREEMPTIVE TREATMENT/LATENT INFECTION TREATMENT ("PROPHYLAXIS OF SYMPTOMATIC INFECTION")

Tuberculosis (latent tuberculosis infection, defined by a positive skin test or IGRA, with no clinical or x-ray evidence of active disease)	INH 10–15 mg/kg/day (max 300 mg) PO daily for 9 mo (12 mo for immunocompromised patients) (AIII); treatment with INH at 20–30 mg twice weekly for 9 mo is also effective (AIII)	Single drug therapy if no clinical or radiographic evidence of active disease. For exposure to known INH-R but rifampin-S strains, use rifampin 6 mo (AIII). For exposure to multidrug-resistant strains, consult with TB specialist.

D. SURGICAL/PROCEDURE PROPHYLAXIS

The CDC and National Healthcare Safety Network use a classification of surgical procedure-related wound infections based on an estimation of the load of bacterial contamination: Class I, clean; Class II, clean-contaminated; Class III, contaminated; and Class IV, dirty-infected.Other major factors creating risk for postoperative surgical site infection include the duration of surgery (a longer duration operation, defined as one that exceeded the 75th percentile for a given procedure) and the medical comorbidities of the patient, as determined by an American Society of Anesthesiology score of III, IV or V (presence of severe systemic disease that results in functional limitations, is life-threatening, or is expected to preclude survival from the operation). The virulence/pathogenicity of bacteria inoculated and the presence of foreign debris/devitalized tissue/surgical material in the wound are also considered risk factors for infection.

For all categories of surgical prophylaxis, dosing recommendations are based on (1) choosing agents based on the organisms likely to be responsible for wound infections at the surgical site; (2) giving the agents shortly before starting the operation to achieve appropriate serum and tissue exposures at the time of incision through the end of the procedure; (3) providing additional doses during the procedure at times based on the standard dosing guideline for that agent; and (4) stopping the agents at the end of the procedure, but no longer than 24 to 48 hours after the procedure.

Procedure/Operation	Recommended Agents	Preoperative Dose
Cardiovascular		
Cardiothoracic S epidermidis, S aureus, Corynebacterium sp	Cefazolin, OR	25 mg/kg
	Vancomycin (if MRSA or MRSE is likely)	10 mg/kg
Vascular S epidermidis, S aureus, Corynebacterium sp, gram-negative enteric bacilli, particularly for procedures in the groin	Cefazolin, OR	25 mg/kg
	Vancomycin (if MRSA or MRSE is likely)	10 mg/kg

D. SURGICAL/PROCEDURE PROPHYLAXIS (cont)

Procedure/Operation	Recommended Agents	Preoperative Dose
Gastrointestinal		
Gastroduodenal Enteric gram-negative bacilli, respiratory tract gram-positive cocci	Cefazolin, OR	25 mg/kg
	Cefoxitin	40 mg/kg
Biliary Procedure, Open Enteric gram-negative bacilli, enterococci, *Clostridia*	Cefazolin, OR	25 mg/kg
	Cefoxitin	40 mg/kg
Appendectomy, non-perforated	Cefoxitin, OR	40 mg/kg
	Cefazolin and metronidazole	25 mg/kg cefazolin and 10 mg/kg metronidazole
Complicated appendicitis or other ruptured viscus Enteric gram-negative bacilli, enterococci, anaerobes. May require additional therapy for treatment of infection.	Cefoxitin, OR	40 mg/kg
	Cefazolin and metronidazole, OR	25 mg/kg cefazolin and 10 mg/kg metronidazole
	Meropenem, OR	20 mg/kg
	Imipenen, OR	20 mg/kg
	Ertapenem	30 mg/kg
Genitourinary		
Cystoscopy (only requires prophylaxis for children with suspected active UTI, or those having foreign material placed) Enteric gram-negative bacilli, enterococci	Cefazolin, OR	25 mg/kg
	TMP/SMX	4–5 mg/kg
Open or laparoscopic surgery Enteric gram-negative bacilli, enterococci	Cefazolin	25 mg/kg

Head and Neck Surgery		
Assuming incision through oral or pharyngeal mucosa Anaerobes, enteric gram-negative bacilli, S aureus	Clindamycin	10 mg/kg
	Cefazolin and metronidazole	25 mg/kg cefazolin and 10 mg/kg metronidazole
Neurosurgery		
Craniotomy, ventricular shunt placement S epidermidis, S aureus	Cefazolin, OR	25 mg/kg
	Vancomycin, if MRSA or MRSE is likely	10 mg/kg
Orthopedic		
Internal fixation of fractures, spinal rod placement, prosthetic joints S epidermidis, S aureus	Cefazolin, OR	25 mg/kg
	Vancomycin, if MRSA or MRSE is likely	10 mg/kg
Trauma		
Exceptionally varied; agents should focus on skin flora (S epidermidis, S aureus) as well as the flora inoculated into the wound, based on the trauma exposure, that may include enteric gram-negative bacilli, anaerobes (including Clostridia sp), fungi. Cultures at time of wound exploration are critical to focus therapy.	Cefazolin (for skin) OR	25 mg/kg
	Vancomycin (for skin)	10 mg/kg
	Meropenem or imipenem (for anaerobes, including Clostridia sp, and non-fermenting gram-negative bacilli) OR	20 mg/kg for either
	Gentamicin and metronidazole (for anaerobes, including Clostridia sp, and non-fermenting gram-negative bacilli)	2.5 mg/kg (gentamicin) and 10 mg/kg (metronidazole)

15. Sequential Parenteral-Oral Antibiotic Therapy (Oral Step-Down Therapy) for Serious Infections

Bacterial pneumonias, bone and joint infections, deep-tissue abscesses, and appendicitis often require prolonged antibiotic therapy. Many other infections, such as cellulitis or pyelonephritis, may require initial parenteral therapy to control the growth and spread of pathogens. However, intravenous (IV) therapy carries risks of catheter-related complications that are unpleasant for the child whether therapy is provided in the hospital or on an outpatient basis. For the beta-lactam class of antibiotics, absorption of orally administered antibiotics in standard dosages provides peak serum concentrations that are only 5% to 10% of those achieved with IV or intramuscular administration. However, clindamycin and many newer antibiotics of the fluoroquinolone (ciprofloxacin) and oxazolidinone (linezolid) class have excellent absorption of their oral formulations and provide virtually the same tissue antibiotic exposure at a particular mg/kg dose, compared with the exposure when the antibiotic is given at that dose IV. Following initial parenteral therapy of serious infections, it may be possible to provide oral antibiotic therapy to achieve the tissue antibiotic exposure that is required for cure. One must also assume that the parent and child are compliant with the administration of each antibiotic dose, and that the parents will seek medical care if the clinical course does not continue to improve for their child.

High-dose oral beta-lactam antibiotic therapy of osteoarticular infections, associated with achieving a particular level of bactericidal activity in serum, has been associated with treatment success since 1978. While most hospital laboratories no longer offer bactericidal assays, the need to achieve bactericidal activity with high-dose oral therapy, explained below, remains important. Comparable mg/kg dosages of parenteral and oral beta lactam medications often result in comparable tissue concentrations 4 to 6 hours after a dose. The momentary high serum concentrations that occur during IV administration of beta-lactam antibiotics may provide for better tissue penetration, but killing of bacteria by beta-lactam antibiotics is not dependent on the height of the antibiotic concentration, but on the time that the antibiotic is present at the site of infection at concentrations above the minimum inhibitory concentrations.

For abscesses in soft tissues, joints, and bones, most organisms are removed by surgical drainage and killed by the initial parenteral therapy. When the signs and symptoms of infection begin to resolve, usually within 3 to 5 days, continuing IV therapy may not be required as a normal host response begins to assist in clearing the infection.

Large dosage oral beta-lactam therapy (based on in vitro susceptibilities) provides the tissue antibiotic exposure required to eradicate remaining pathogens as the tissue perfusion improves. Begin with a dosage 2 to 3 times the normal dosage (eg, 75–100 mg/kg/day of dicloxacillin or 100 mg/kg/day of cephalexin). High-dose prolonged oral beta-lactam therapy may be associated with reversible neutropenia; checking for hematologic toxicity every few weeks during therapy should be considered.

For methicillin-resistant *Staphylococcus aureus* infections, prospective evaluations of clindamycin or trimethoprim/sulfamethoxazole have not been conducted, but data on clindamycin for osteomyelitis were published decades ago. Dose-limiting diarrhea prevents increasing the dose above 30 to 40 mg/kg/day, divided 3 times daily.

Monitor the child clinically for a continued response on oral therapy; follow C-reactive protein concentrations and erythrocyte sedimentation rate to make sure that the infection is continuing to respond to the antibiotic and dosage you selected.

16. Adverse Reactions to Antimicrobial Agents

A good rule of clinical practice is to be suspicious of an adverse drug reaction when a patient's clinical course deviates from the expected. This section focuses on reactions that may require close observation or laboratory monitoring either because of their frequency or because of their severity. For more detailed listings of reactions, review the US Food and Drug Administration (FDA)-approved package labels or reference texts (such as *AHFS Drug Information 2009*, American Society of Hospital Pharmacists, Inc., Bethesda, MD). In addition, FDA-approved package labels for most drugs can be accessed online at the National Library of Medicine (NLM) site, with information from the FDA at http:// dailymed.nlm.nih.gov/dailymed/about.cfm. For many of the more recently approved antibiotics, adverse reaction rates in both antibiotic- and comparator-treated populations are provided to allow you to draw your own conclusions about safety and the risk of adverse reactions. The NLM provides an online drug information service (Medline Plus), accessed at http://www.nlm.nih.gov/medlineplus/ druginformation.html.

Antibacterial Drugs
Aminoglycosides
Any of the aminoglycosides can cause serious nephrotoxicity and ototoxicity. Monitor all patients receiving aminoglycoside therapy for more than a few days for renal function with periodic determinations of blood urea nitrogen and creatinine to assess potential problems of drug accumulation with deteriorating renal function. Common practice is to measure the peak serum concentration 0.5 to 1.0 hour after a dose to make sure one is in a safe and therapeutic range and to measure a trough serum concentration immediately preceding a dose to assess for drug accumulation and pending toxicity. Monitoring is especially important in patients with any degree of renal insufficiency. Elevated trough concentrations (>2 mg/mL for gentamicin and tobramycin, and >10 mg/mL for amikacin) suggest drug accumulation and should be a warning to decrease the dose, even if the peak is not yet elevated. Renal toxicity may be related to the total exposure of the kidney to the aminoglycoside over time. With once-daily administration regimens, peak values are 2 to 3 times greater, and trough values are usually very low. Nephrotoxicity seems to be less common in adults with once-daily (as opposed to 3 times daily) dosing regimens; but data are lacking in children.

The "loop" diuretics (furosemide and bumetanide) potentiate the ototoxicity of the aminoglycosides. Aminoglycosides potentiate botulinum toxin and are to be avoided in young infants with infant botulism.

The aminoglycosides are well tolerated via intramuscular and intravenous (IV) routes of administration. Minor side effects, such as allergies, rashes, and drug fever, are rare.

Beta-Lactam Antibiotics
The most feared reaction to penicillins, anaphylactic shock, is extremely rare, and no absolutely reliable means of predicting its occurrence exists. For most infections, alternative therapy to penicillin or beta-lactams exists. However, in certain situations, the benefits of penicillin or a beta-lactam may outweigh the risk of anaphylaxis, requiring that skin testing and desensitization be performed in a medically supervised environment. The commercially available skin testing material, benzylpenicilloyl polylysine (Pre Pen, AllerQuest) was approved and marketed in September 2009. It contains the major determinants thought to be primarily responsible for urticarial reactions, but does not contain the minor determinants that are more often associated with anaphylaxis. No commercially available

minor determinant mixture is available. Some authorities use a dilute solution of freshly prepared benzyl penicillin G as the skin test material in place of a standardized mixture of minor determinants. Testing should be performed on children with a credible history of a possible reaction to a penicillin before these drugs are used in either oral or parenteral formulations. Anaphylaxis has been reported in adults receiving penicillin skin testing. A recent review provides a more in-depth discussion, with additional information on desensitization available at the Centers for Disease Control and Prevention Web site (www.cdc.gov/STD/treatment/2006/penicillin-allergy.htm#skintesting). Cross-reactions between classes of beta-lactam antibiotics (penicillins, cephalosporins, carbapenems, and monobactams) occur at a rate of between 5% to 20%. No commercially available skin testing reagent has been developed for beta-lactam antibiotics other than penicillin.

Amoxicillin and other aminopenicillins are associated with minor adverse effects. Diarrhea, oral or diaper area candidiasis, morbilliform, and blotchy rashes are not uncommon. The kinds of non-urticarial rashes that may occur while a child is receiving amoxicillin are not known to predispose to anaphylaxis and may not actually be caused by amoxicillin itself; they do not represent a routine contraindication to subsequent use of amoxicillin or any other penicillins. Rarely, beta-lactams cause serious, life-threatening pseudomembranous enterocolitis due to suppression of normal bowel flora and overgrowth of toxin-producing strains of *Clostridium difficile*. Drug-related fever may occur; serum sickness is uncommon. Reversible neutropenia and thrombocytopenia may occur with any of the beta-lactams and seem to be related to dose and duration of therapy.

The cephalosporins have been a remarkably safe series of antibiotics. The third-generation cephalosporins cause profound alteration of normal flora on mucosal surfaces, and all have caused pseudomembranous colitis on rare occasions. Ceftriaxone commonly causes loose stools, but it is rarely severe enough to require stopping therapy. Ceftriaxone in high dosages may cause fine "sand" (a calcium complex of ceftriaxone) to develop in the gallbladder. In adults, and rarely in children, these deposits may cause biliary tract symptoms; these are not gallstones, and the deposits are reversible after stopping the drug. In neonates receiving calcium-containing hyperalimentation concurrent with IV ceftriaxone, precipitation of ceftriaxone-calcium in the bloodstream resulting in death has been reported, leading to an FDA warning against the concurrent use of ceftriaxone and parenteral calcium in infants younger than 28 days (http://www.fda.gov/Drugs/DrugSafetyPostmarketDrugSafety InformationforPatientsandProviders/ucm109103.htm). As ceftriaxone may also displace bilirubin from albumin-binding sites and increase free bilirubin in serum, the antibiotic is not routinely used in neonatal infections until the normal physiologic jaundice is resolving after the first few weeks of life. Cefotaxime is the preferred IV third-generation cephalosporin for neonates.

Imipenem-cilastatin, meropenem, and ertapenem have rates of adverse effects on hematopoietic, hepatic, and renal systems that are similar to other beta-lactams. However, children treated with imipenem for bacterial meningitis were noted to have an increase in probable drug-related seizures not seen with meropenem therapy in controlled studies. For children requiring carbapenem therapy, meropenem is preferred for those with any underlying central nervous system inflammatory condition.

Fluoroquinolones (FQs)
All quinolone antibiotics (nalidixic acid, ciprofloxacin, levofloxacin, gatifloxacin, and moxifloxacin) cause cartilage damage to weight-bearing joints in toxicity studies in various

immature animals; however, no conclusive data indicate similar toxicity in young children. Studies to evaluate cartilage toxicity and failure to achieve predicted growth have not consistently found statistically significant differences between those children treated with FQs and controls, although in an FDA-requested, blinded, prospective study of complicated urinary tract infections, the number of muscular/joint/tendon events was greater in the ciprofloxacin-treated group than in the comparator (http://www.fda.gov/downloads/Drugs/DevelopmentApproval Process/DevelopmentResources/UCM162536.pdf). This continues to be an area of active investigation by the pediatric infectious diseases community as well as the FDA. Fluoroquinolone toxicities in adults, which vary in incidence considerably between individual agents, include cardiac dysrhythmias, hepatotoxicity, and photodermatitis; other reported side effects include gastrointestinal symptoms, dizziness, headaches, tremors, confusion, seizures, and alterations of glucose metabolism producing both hyper- and hypoglycemia.

Lincosamides

Clindamycin can cause nausea, vomiting, and diarrhea. Pseudomembranous colitis due to suppression of normal flora and overgrowth of *C difficile* is uncommon, especially in children, but potentially serious. Urticaria, glossitis, pruritus, and skin rashes occur occasionally. Serum sickness, anaphylaxis, and photosensitivity are rare, as are hematologic and hepatic abnormalities. Extensive use of clindamycin since 2000 for treatment of community-associated methicillin-resistant *Staphylococcus aureus* infections has not been accompanied by reports of increasing rates of *C difficile*–mediated colitis in children.

Macrolides

Erythromycin is one of the safest antimicrobial agents. However, it commonly produces nausea and epigastric distress. Azithromycin and clarithromycin cause fewer gastrointestinal side effects than erythromycin. Alteration of normal flora is generally not a problem, but oral or perianal candidiasis occasionally develops. Transient cholestatic hepatitis is a rare complication that occurs with approximately equal frequency among the various formulations of erythromycin. Intravenous erythromycin lactobionate causes phlebitis and should be administered slowly (1–2 hours), the gastrointestinal side effects seen with oral administration also accompany IV use. However, IV azithromycin is better tolerated than IV erythromycin, and has been evaluated for pharmacokinetics in limited numbers of children.

Erythromycin therapy has been associated with pyloric stenosis in newborns and young infants; due to this toxicity and with limited data on safety of azithromycin in the first months of life, azithromycin is now the preferred macrolide for treatment of pertussis in neonates and young infants.

Oxazolidinones

Linezolid represents the first oxazolidinone antibiotic approved for all children, including neonates, by the FDA. Toxicity is primarily hematologic, with thrombocytopenia and neutropenia that is dependent on dosage and duration of therapy, occurring most often with treatment courses of 2 weeks or longer. Routine monitoring for bone marrow toxicity every 1 to 2 weeks is recommended for children on long-term therapy. Peripheral neuropathy and optic neuritis may also occur with long-term therapy.

Sulfonamides and Trimethoprim

The most common adverse reaction to sulfonamides is a hypersensitivity rash, which occurs much more commonly in children with HIV infection on therapy. The frequency and types of reactions to the trimpethoprim/sulfamethoxazole (TMP/SMX) combination are said to be the same as with sulfamethoxazole alone, but it is not clear whether the most significant reaction, Stevens-Johnson syndrome, is caused more often by the combination than by sulfamethoxazole alone. Neutropenia and anemia occur occasionally. Mild depression of platelet counts occurs in approximately one-half the patients treated with sulfas or TMP/SMX, and seems to be dosage-related, but this rarely produces clinical bleeding problems. Sulfa drugs can precipitate hemolysis in patients with glucose-6-phosphate dehydrogenase deficiency. Drug fever and serum sickness are infrequent hypersensitivity reactions. Hepatitis with focal or diffuse necrosis is rare. A rare idiosyncratic reaction to sulfa drugs is acute aseptic meningitis.

Tetracyclines

Tetracyclines are used infrequently in pediatric patients because the major indications are uncommon diseases (rickettsial infections, brucellosis, Lyme disease), with the exception of acne. Side effects include minor gastrointestinal disturbances, photosensitization, angioedema, browning of the tongue, glossitis, pruritus ani, and exfoliative dermatitis. Potential adverse drug reactions from tetracyclines involve virtually every organ system. Hepatic and pancreatic injuries have occurred with accidental overdosage and in patients with renal failure. (Pregnant women are particularly at risk for hepatic injury.) Tetracyclines are deposited in growing bones and teeth, with depression of linear bone growth, dental staining, and defects in enamelization in deciduous and permanent teeth. This effect is dose-related, and the risk extends up to 8 years of age. A single treatment course of tetracyclines has not been found to cause dental staining, leading to the recommendation for tetracyclines as the drugs of choice in children for a number of uncommon pathogens. A new parenteral tetracycline approved for adults in 2005, tigecycline, produces the same "staining" of bones in experimental animals as seen with previous tetracyclines.

Vancomycin

Vancomycin can cause phlebitis if the drug is injected rapidly or in concentrated form. Vancomycin has the potential for ototoxicity and nephrotoxicity, and serum concentrations should be monitored for children on more than a few days of therapy. Hepatic toxicity is rare. Neutropenia has been reported. If the drug is infused too rapidly, a transient rash of the upper body with itching may occur from histamine release (red man syndrome). It is not a contraindication to continued use and the rash is less likely to occur if the infusion rate is increased to 60 to 120 minutes and the children are pretreated with oral or IV antihistamines.

Antituberculous Drugs

Isoniazid (INH) is generally well tolerated and hypersensitivity reactions are rare. Peripheral neuritis (preventable or reversed by pyridoxine administration) and mental aberrations from euphoria to psychosis occur more often in adults than in children. Mild elevations of alanine transaminase in the first weeks of therapy, which disappear or remain stable with continued administration, are common. Rarely, hepatitis develops, but is reversible if INH is stopped; if INH is not stopped, liver failure may develop in these children. Monitoring of liver functions is not routinely required in children receiving INH single drug therapy for latent tuberculosis as long as the children can be followed closely and liver functions can be drawn if the child develops symptoms of hepatitis.

Rifampin can also cause hepatitis; it is more common in patients with preexisting liver disease or in those taking large dosages. The risk of hepatic damage increases when rifampin and INH are taken together in dosages of more than 15 mg/kg/day of each. Gastrointestinal, hematologic, and neurologic side effects of various types have been observed on occasion. Hypersensitivity reactions are rare.

Pyrazinamide also can cause hepatic damage, which again seems to be dosage-related. Ethambutol has the potential for optic neuritis, but this toxicity seems to be rare in children at currently prescribed dosages, and routine screening for color vision is no longer recommended.

Antifungal Drugs

Amphotericin B (deoxycholate) causes chills, fever, flushing, and headaches, the most common of the many adverse reactions. Some degree of decreased renal function occurs in virtually all patients given amphotericin B. Anemia is common and, rarely, hepatic toxicity and neutropenia occur. Patients should be monitored for hyponatremia and hypokalemia. However, much better tolerated (but more costly) lipid formulations of amphotericin B are now commonly used (see Chapter 2). For reasons of safety and tolerability, the lipid formulations should be used whenever possible.

Ketoconazole produces hepatic damage on rare occasions. The most common side effect is gastric distress; this can often be alleviated by dividing the daily dose. Gynecomastia is not rare in adult males. Itraconazole has a smaller incidence of adverse effects than ketoconazole.

Fluconazole is usually very well tolerated from both clinical and laboratory standpoints. Gastrointestinal symptoms, rash, and headache occur occasionally. Transient, asymptomatic elevations of hepatic enzymes have been reported but are rare.

Voriconazole, a new antifungal suspension, may interfere with metabolism of other drugs the child may be receiving due to hepatic P450 metabolism. However, a poorly understood visual field abnormality has been described, usually at the beginning of a course of therapy, and uniformly self-resolving, in which objects appear to glow. There is no pain and no known anatomic or biochemical correlate of this side effect; no lasting effects on vision have yet been reported. Hepatic toxicity has also been reported, but is not so common as to preclude the use of voriconazole for serious fungal infections.

Caspofungin is very well tolerated, is now FDA approved for use in children down to 3 months of age, and has minimal side effects. Fever, rash, headache, and phlebitis at the site of infection have been reported in adults. Uncommon hepatic side effects have also been reported. Micafungin and anidulofungin seem to have the same benign side effect profile in adults as caspofungin. Neither of these 2 echinocandins is well studied in children.

Flucytosine (5-FC) is seldom used due to the availability of safer, equally effective therapy. The major toxicity is bone marrow depression, which is dosage related, especially in patients treated concomitantly with amphotericin B. Renal function should be monitored.

Antiviral Drugs

After extensive clinical use, acyclovir has proved to be a safe drug with rare serious adverse effects. Renal dysfunction with IV acyclovir has occurred mainly with too rapid infusion of the drug. Rash, headache, and gastrointestinal side effects are uncommon. There has been little controlled experience in children with famciclovir and valacyclovir.

Ganciclovir causes hematologic toxicity that is dependent on the dosage and duration of therapy. Gastrointestinal disturbances and neurologic damage are rarely encountered.

Amantadine produces dizziness, drowsiness, and insomnia in many patients, but these effects are usually not severe. Rimantadine has fewer side effects. Visual disturbances, confusion, and psychosis are rare.

Oseltamivir is well tolerated except for nausea with or without vomiting, which may be more likely to occur with the first few doses, but usually resolves within a few days while still on therapy. Neuropsychiatric events have been reported, primarily from Japan, in patients with influenza treated with oseltamivir (a rate of approximately 1:50,000). These adverse events have not been reported in patients taking oseltamivir prophylaxis. Based on an FDA assessment (which is ongoing), it seems that these spontaneously reported side effects may be a function of influenza itself, oseltamivir itself, possibly a genetic predisposition to this clinical event, or a combination of all 3.

Foscarnet can cause renal dysfunction, anemia, and cardiac rhythm disturbances. Seizures and neuropathy are other serious but rare toxicities.

The many antiviral drugs for treatment for HIV infection have many adverse effects; consult the current FDA-approved package labels.

17. Drug Interactions

NOTES

- Antimicrobial drug-drug interactions that are known to be or have the potential to be clinically significant in children are listed in this chapter. Interactions involving probenecid, synergy-antagonism, and physical incompatibilities are not listed. Interactions involving antiretrovirals can be found at http://aidsinfo.nih.gov/contentfiles/PediatricGuidelines.pdf. Citations at the end of this section provide more extensive details of all reported and theoretical interactions, including antimicrobial drug-disease interactions.
- **Abbreviations:** ACE, angiotensin-converting enzyme; Conc, concentration; Decr, decreased; EIAED, enzyme-inducing antiepileptic drugs; FQs, fluoroquinolones; Incr, increased; MAO, monoamine oxidase; Poss, possible; NSAID, nonsteroidal anti-inflammatory drug; PPI, proton pump inhibitors; SRI, serotonin reuptake inhibitors; TMP/SMX, trimethoprim/sulfamethoxazole.

Anti-infective Agent	Interacting Drug(s)	Adverse Effect
Acyclovir/valacyclovir	Nephrotoxins[a]	Additive nephrotoxicity
	Phenytoin, valproic acid	Decr seizure control
Albendazole	EIAED[b]	Decr conc of albendazole
Amantadine	Anticholinergics[c]	Additive anticholinergic toxicity
	Bupropion	Additive neurotoxicity
	Trimethoprim	Incr amantadine conc
Amikacin	(See Aminoglycosides[d])	
Aminoglycosides[d] (parenteral)	Nephrotoxins[a]	Additive nephrotoxicity
	Neuromuscular blocking agents	Incr neuromuscular blockade
	Indomethacin, ibuprofen	Incr aminoglycoside conc Additive nephrotoxicity
	Carbo-/cisplatin, ethacrynic acid	Additive ototoxicity
Amphotericin B	Nephrotoxins[a]	Additive nephrotoxicity
	Cisplatin, corticosteroids, diuretics	Additive hypokalemia
Atovaquone	Metoclopramide, rifamycins, tetracyline	Decr atovaquone conc
Carbapenems	Valproic acid	Decr conc of valproic acid

Anti-infective Agent	Interacting Drug(s)	Adverse Effect
Caspofungin	Cyclosporine	Transient elevated hepatic
	Tacrolimus, sirolimus	Decr tacrolimus/sirolimus conc
	Rifampin, EIAED[b]	Decr caspofungin conc
Cefaclor, cefdinir, cefpodoxime, cefuroxime (oral)	Antacids, H2 antagonists[e], PPI[f]	Decr antibiotic conc
Ceftriaxone	Calcium intravenous	Precipitation, cardiopulmonary embolism
Chloramphenicol[g]	Phenytoin, PPI[f], sulfonylureas	Incr conc of interacting drug
	EIAED[b], rifamycins	Decr chloramphenicol conc
Cidofovir	Nephrotoxins[a]	Additive nephrotoxicty
Ciprofloxacin[h]	Caffeine, clozapine, diazepam, duloxetine, glyburide, methadone, olanzapine, sildenafil, theophylline, warfarin	Incr conc of interacting drug
	Phenytoin	Incr or decr conc of phenytoin
	Foscarnet	Additive seizure toxicity
	Antacids, bismuth, calcium, iron, sucralfate, zinc	Decr oral absorption
Clarithromycin[g]	(See Erythromycin.)	
Clindamycin	Neuromuscular blocking agents	Incr neuromuscular blockade
Dapsone	Rifampin	Decr dapsone conc
Daptomycin	Statins	Additive myopathy
Doxycycline	Antacids, bismuth, calcium, iron, magnesium, sucralfate, zinc	Decr oral absorption
	EIAED[b], rifamycins	Decr doxycycline conc
Erythromycin[g]	Theophylline	Incr conc of interacting drug
	Class IA and III antiarrhythmics, doxapram, droperidol, haloperidol, methadone, pimozide, FQs[h], ziprasidone	Additive arrhythmic cardiotoxicity
	Azole antifungals, diltiazem, verapamil	Incr macrolide conc
	Rifamycins	Decr macrolide conc

Anti-infective Agent	Interacting Drug(s)	Adverse Effect
Fluconazole[g]	Celecoxib, ibuprofen, irbesartan, naproxen, fluvastatin, phenytoin, sulfonylureas, warfarin	Incr conc of interacting drug-CYP 2C9 inhibition
	Losartan	Decr losartan activity
	Rifampin	Decr fluconazole conc
Foscarnet	Pentamidine	Hypocalcemia
	Ciprofloxacin	Additive seizure toxicity
	Nephrotoxins[a]	Additive nephrotoxicty
Ganciclovir/valganciclovir	Imipenem	Additive seizure toxicity
	Hemotoxins[i]	Additive hemotoxicity
	Nephrotoxins[a]	Additive nephrotoxicity
Gentamicin	(See Aminoglycosides[d].)	
Griseofulvin	EIAED[b]	Decr griseofulvin conc
Imipenem	Cyclosporine, ganciclovir	Additive neurotoxicity
Isoniazid[j]	Acetaminophen, carbamazepine	Hepatotoxicity
	Cycloserine	Dizziness, drowsiness
	Carbamazepine, valproate	Incr conc of interacting drug
	Atomoxetine, linezolid	Poss MAO inhibition toxicity
	Amphetamines, buspirone, mirtazipine, SRI[k] tramadol	Poss serotonin syndrome
Itraconazole, ketoconazole	Aripiprazole, benzodiazepines[l] buspirone, busulfan, calcium-channel blockers[m], carbamazepine, chlorpheniramine, corticosteroids, cyclophosphamide, cyclosporine, digoxin, ergotamine, fentanyl, fexofenadine, fluoxetine, haloperidol, loperamide, methadone, pimozide, quetiapine quinidine, rifabutin, sertraline, sildenafil, sirolimus, statins[n], tacrolimus, trazodone, vinca alkaloids, warfarin, zolpidem	Incr conc of interacting drug-CYP 3A4-7 inhibition
	Antacids, H2 antagonists[e] PPI[f] sucralfate	Decr azole conc, itraconazole oral solution less affected
	EIAED[b] rifamycins	Decr azole conc
	Erythromycin, quinolones, ziprasodone	Incr conc of interacting drugs with poss incr cardiotoxicity
	Loratadine, haloperidol, phenytoin	Incr conc of interacting drug

Anti-infective Agent	Interacting Drug(s)	Adverse Effect
Levofloxacin[h]	See Ciprofloxacin for drugs that decr oral absorption of FQ.	
Linezolid	Atomoxetine, isoniazid	Poss MAO inhibition toxicity
	Sympathomimetics	Poss hypertension
	Amphetamines, buspirone, mirtazipine, SRI[k] tramadol	Poss serotonin syndrome
Metronidazole	Amiodarone, busulfan, carbamazepine, cyclosporine, 5-fluorouacil, lithium, phenytoin, tacrolimus, warfarin	Incr conc of interacting drug
	EIAED[b]	Decr metronidazole conc
Micafungin	Cyclosporine, sirolimus	Incr conc of interacting drug
Minocycline	Antacids, bismuth, calcium, iron, magnesium, sucralfate, zinc	Decr oral absorption
Nafcillin	Cyclosporine	± cyclosporine conc
	Calcium channel blockers[m]	Decr conc of interacting drug
	Warfarin	Warfarin resistance
Norfloxacin	Cyclosporine	Incr cyclosporine conc
	See Ciprofloxacin for drugs that decr oral absorption of FQ.	
Penicillins	Methotrexate	Incr methotrexate conc
Posaconazole[g]	Phenytoin	Decr conc of posaconazole
Praziquantel	EIAED[b]	Decr conc of praziquantel
Quinupristin/dalfopristin[g]	(See Itraconazole for list of interacting drugs.)	
Rifampin, Rifabutin	Numerous including: amiodarone, anticonvulsants, antidepressants, antipsychotics, barbiturates, benzodiazepines[j], beta-adrenergic blockers, buspirone, coxibs, calcium channel blockers[m], oral contraceptives, corticosteroids, digoxin, immunosuppressants, NSAIDs, opioids, statins, sulfonylureas, warfarin, zolpidem	Decr conc of interacting drug See also *Clinical Pharmacokinetics* 2003;42(9):819–850.
Streptomycin	(See Aminoglycosides[d].)	
Telithromycing	(See Erythromycin.)	
Terbinafine	Most SRI[k], tricyclic antidepressants	Incr conc of interacting drug
	Rifampin	Decr terbinafine conc

Anti-infective Agent	Interacting Drug(s)	Adverse Effect
Tetracycline	Antacids, bismuth, calcium, iron, magnesium, sucralfate, zinc	Decr oral absorption
	Atovaquone	Decr atovaquone conc
	Isotretinoin	Additive intracranial hypertension
TMP/SMX	Cyclosporine, losartan	Decr conc of interacting drug
	Azathioprine, methotrexate	Additive hematological toxicity
	Rifamycins	Decr TMP/SMX conc
	Celecoxib, dapsone, digoxin, dofetilide, fluoxetine, fluvastatin, methotrexate, NSAIDs, phenytoin, procainamide, sulfonylureas, voriconazole, warfarin	Incr conc of interacting drug
	ACE Inhibitors, spironolactone	Hyperkalemia
Tobramycin	(See Aminoglycosides[d].)	
Vancomycin	Indomethacin, ibuprofen	Incr vancomycin conc
Voriconazole[g,j]	Methadone, omeprazole	Incr conc of interacting drug
	EIAED[b], rifamycins	Decr voriconazole conc

[a] Potentially nephrotoxic drugs include aminoglycosides, acyclovir, cidofovir, ganciclovir, foscarnet, ACE inhibitors, cyclosporine, diuretics, NSAIDs, contrast agents, pentamidine, tacrolimus, tenofovir.

[b] EIAED: carbamazepine, phenobarbital, phenytoin, and primidone.

[c] Examples of anticholinergics: atropine, belladonna, benztropine, clidinium, dicyclomine, diphenhydramine, glycopyrrolate, homatropine, hyoscyamine, promethazine, propantheline, scopolamine.

[d] Gentamicin, tobramycin, amikacin, streptomycin.

[e] Famotidine, ranitidine.

[f] Pantoprazole, rabeprazole, omeprazole, lansoprazole, esomeprazole.

[g] Antibiotic is known to have or may potentially have the same interactions as itraconazole due to similar inhibition of CYP3A4-7 drug metabolism.

[h] FQs as a class have dose- and drug-dependant cardiac QTc interval prolongation effects. When used with other drugs that share this cardiac effect, there may be an additive cardiotoxic interaction. Ciprofloxacin and levofloxacin are FQs sometimes used in children; their risk of prolonging the QTc interval is low compared to other FQs.

[i] Notable hemotoxic drugs include antineoplastics, clozapine, dapsone, flucytosine, mycophenolate, pentamidine, primaquine, pyrimethaine, TMP/SMX, zidovudine.

[j] Antibiotic is known to have or may potentially have the same interactions as fluconazole due to similar inhibition of CYP2C9 drug metabolism.

[k] SRI: buproprion, citalopram, duloxetine, escitalopram, fluoxetine, fluvoxamine, nefazodone, paroxetine, sertraline, venlafaxine.

[l] CYP3A4 oxidized benzodiazepines: alprazolam, chlordiazepoxide, clonazepam, clorazepate, diazepam, midazolam, and triazolam.

[m] Amlodipine, bepridil, diltiazem, felodipine, isradipine, nicardipine, nifedipine, nimodipine, verapamil.

[n] Atorvastatin, lovastatin, simvastatin

Bibliography

Allegaert K, Rayyan M, Anderson BJ. Impact of ibuprofen administration on renal drug clearance in the first weeks of life. *Methods Find Exp Clin Pharmacol.* 2006;28(8):519–522

Baxter K. *Stockley's Drug Interactions.* 8th ed. Chicago, IL: Pharmaceutical Press; 2008

Bradley JS, Wassel RT, Lee L, Nambiar S. Intravenous ceftriaxone and calcium in the neonate: assessing the risk for cardiopulmonary adverse events. *Pediatrics.* 2009;123(4):e609–e613

Bruggemann RJ, Alffenaar JW, Blijlevens NM. Clinical relevance of the pharmacokinetic interactions of azole antifungal drugs with other coadministered agents. *Clin Infect Dis.* 2009;48(10):1441–1458

Flockhart DA. Cytochrome P450 drug interaction table. *Drug Interactions.* http://medicine.iupui.edu/flockhart. Accessed August 2009.

Gubbins PO, Amsden JR. Drug-drug interactions of antifungal agents and implications for patient care. *Expert Opin Pharmacother.* 2005;6(13):2231–2243

Hansten PD, Horn JR. *Hansten and Horn's Drug Interactions, Analysis and Management.* 4th ed. Philadelphia, PA: Lippincott Wilkins & Williams; 2009

Pai MP, Momary KM, Rodvold KA. Antibiotic drug interactions. *Med Clin North Am.* 2006;90(6):1223–1255

Perucca E. Clinically relevant drug interactions with antiepileptic drugs. *Br J Clin Pharmacol.* 2006;61(3):246–255

Piscitelli, SC, Rodvold KA. *Drug Interactions in Infectious Diseases.* 2nd ed. Totowa, NJ: Humana Press; 2005

Simkó J, Csilek A, Karászi J, Lorincz I. Proarrhythmic potential of antimicrobial agents. *Infection.* 2008;36(3):194–206

Appendix

Nomogram for Determining Body Surface Area

Based on the nomogram shown in Figure C-4, a straight line joining the patient's height and weight will intersect the center column at the calculated body surface area (BSA). For children of normal height and weight, the child's weight in pounds is used, then the examiner reads across to the corresponding BSA in meters. Alternatively, Mosteller's formula can be used.

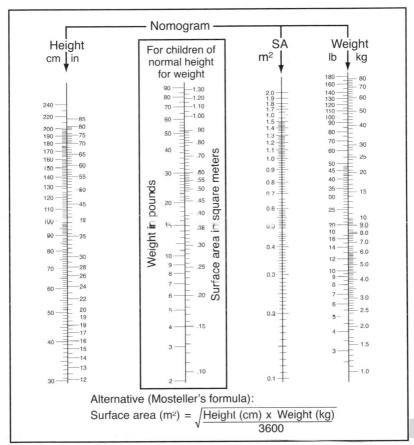

Alternative (Mosteller's formula):

$$\text{Surface area (m}^2) = \sqrt{\frac{\text{Height (cm)} \times \text{Weight (kg)}}{3600}}$$

Nomogram and equation to determine body surface area. (From: Tschudy MM, Arcara KM, eds. *The Harriet Lane Handbook.* 19th ed. St Louis, MO: Mosby; 2012. |Data from Briars GL, Bailey BJ. Surface area estimation: pocket calculator v nomogram. *Arch Dis Child.* 1994;70[3]:246 Reprinted with permission from Elsevier.)

Index